THE HAPPY VEGAN

THE HAPPY VEGAN

A GUIDE TO LIVING A LONG, HEALTHY, AND SUCCESSFUL LIFE

RUSSELL SIMMONS

WITH CHRIS MORROW

Avery
an imprint of Penguin Random House
New York

an imprint of Penguin Random House LLC
375 Hudson Street
New York, New York 10014

Most Avery books are available at special quantity discounts for bulk purchase for sales promotions, premiums, fund-raising, and educational needs. Special books or book excerpts also can be created to fit specific needs. For details, write SpecialMarkets@penguinrandomhouse.com.

ISBN 978-1-59240-932-7

Printed in the United States of America
10 9 8 7 6 5 4 3 2 1

Book design by Elke Sigal

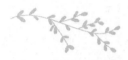

This book is dedicated to the billions of animals who know nothing but horrific abuse and a brutal death. My prayer for this book is that it can help relieve at least some of their suffering, as well as the suffering of Mother Earth and her inhabitants, who are poisoning themselves by ingesting death on a daily basis.

CONTENTS

THE HAPPY VEGAN

All of my books, at their core, have been about the same thing.

How to be happy.

In fact, that mission has been at the heart of everything I've tried to do in my career.

When I wrote *Do You!*, *Super Rich*, and *Success Through Stillness*, it was only to help readers become happier.

Just as when I made records with Def Jam, clothes with Phat Farm, and videos with my latest company, All Def Digital (ADD), it's only been to bring a little more joy into people's lives.

I'm always thrilled when someone comes up to me on the street and says, "Russell, *Do You!* helped me get through a tough time" or "Hearing Run-D.M.C. changed my life!"

It feels great to know that I've contributed, even just a tiny bit, to a positive change in someone's life. But as cool as it has been to get that sort of feedback, I'm expecting a different kind of reaction to this book.

No, *The Happy Vegan* won't just *change* your life.

It can *save* your life. Not to mention save the world as well.

That's a big claim, but it's made with a confidence that can come only from experience. Becoming a vegan hasn't only made me much happier but healthier too. It helped me disconnect from the lifestyle that was making me sick, a lifestyle that has put too many other middle-aged African American males in the ground.

Today, on the verge of my sixth decade, I feel content and centered, full of energy and appetite for all that life has to offer.

I'm in a wonderful space. And I credit much of it to my decision to stop consuming animal products.

It's a space, however, that took a long time to arrive at. As those of you familiar with my story already know, I spent much of the first half of my life abusing my body with various toxins. From weed to coke to angel dust, there wasn't a drug I didn't get high off of. Just as there wasn't a kind of meat or dairy I didn't consume. Products that were, in many ways, just as bad for me as drugs.

I finally got sober at the age of thirty. In my late thirties I embraced the practice of yoga, which helped me leave my toxic lifestyle behind me for good. In literally my first class I experienced a sense of serenity and clarity I'd never felt before. Yoga helped me see that getting high had been nothing but a distraction. I found I preferred waking up sober to going to bed high.

Yoga in turn led me to meditation, which taught me how to further wipe the distractions out of my mind and focus on my best ideas. My personal relationships and business began to improve. Instead of walking around in a daze, I was looking at life through cleaner lenses. It was a great way to live.

Thanks to that clarity, for the first time in my life I also found myself starting to think about the food I was putting into my body. During my yoga classes, my teacher Sharon Gannon (or one of her disciples) would gently but firmly remind us not to put toxins in our bodies. Every day after class, it seemed, I'd meet someone who followed Sharon's mantra and had removed animal products from their diet. Inevitably they were in great shape and smiled a lot. I was impressed. I was also inspired by my great friend (and current head of television development at ADD) Simone Reyes, who had been a vegan for many years. Another big influence was Glen E. Friedman, my senior executive in charge of television development at Def Pictures. Through their collective examples, I felt myself inching closer toward a healthier relationship with the world.

I finally took a great leap forward on New Year's Day 1997. I was staying on the Caribbean island of St. Barts, where I loved (and still love) taking a monthlong vacation during the winter holidays. Glen, as he often does, was staying with me at a villa I'd rented by the island's clear blue ocean.

I woke up New Year's Day planning on hitting the beach, but a peek out the window at the overcast sky told me Mother Nature had other ideas. So Glen and I decided to watch a movie instead.

For months, Glen had been bugging me to watch a film called *Diet for a New America*. Once I watched it, he promised, I'd stop eating animal products and never look back. In my heart I knew he was probably right, just as in my heart I knew the yoga community was right too. I was primed to make a change.

Yet for some reason I'd been resisting watching the tape. Giving up drugs and taking up yoga and meditation had been a major transformation for me. Changing what I ate on top of all that seemed like just a little too much to think about.

Glen is nothing, however, if not determined (it's probably one of the qualities that makes him such a great photographer). He'd brought the film with him to St. Barts in case such a moment would present itself, and now that it had, he wasn't going to miss his chance.

"Russell, stop BSing and let's watch this," he said. "There's nothing else to do today—nobody is going to be on the beach, the stores are closed, and all your friends are sleeping off hangovers. Enough with the excuses. Today's the day."

I knew he was right. "Let's do it," I said.

Glen popped in the VHS tape (remember those?), and I quickly learned that *Diet for a New America* was a PBS special hosted by John Robbins, named after the best-selling book he'd written a couple years earlier. John's father had cofounded the Baskin-Robbins ice cream empire and John had grown up eating a "normal" American diet, heavy on meat and dairy. After a series of illnesses, Robbins took a closer look at his diet. After years of research he came to the conclusion that meat and dairy were actually responsible for many of his health problems. He then dedicated his life to spreading the word about the dangers of consuming animal products.

As the taped rolled, I was struck by Robbins's profiles of men in their thirties and forties who were on the verge of death because of the damage meat and dairy had done to their cardiovascular systems. Men who frankly looked a lot like *me*. A doctor spoke about how one of his patients—a man in his early thirties—dropped dead one night after eating a burger and a milk shake. His body just couldn't take the abuse anymore. That really affected me. I'd had *a lot* of burgers and milk shakes over the years.

I was also shocked to learn the degree to which the meat and dairy industries were responsible for polluting our nation's waterways and contributing to global warming.

Equally powerful were the scenes showing the horrible conditions animals are raised in and the barbaric ways they're slaughtered for their meat. I had always subscribed to the fairy tale that animals lived on farms, grazed in the sun, and ate grass. Watching chickens being thrown into grinders alive, cattle squirming on squalid floors after having their throats slit, and caged pigs desperately trying to reach their piglets, was the rudest of awakenings. After one such scene, Robbins said something that struck me to my core: "As a concerned citizen, as someone who wants my life to be a statement of compassion, when I see what's done to the animals, it makes me look at my food choices in a whole new way. I have to question, is that what I want my contribution to the world to involve?"

The tape rolled on, but Robbins's words had already led me to an epiphany:

No, I *didn't* want to be involved in the torture and slaughter of animals anymore.

No, I *didn't* want to drop dead in my forties from eating too many burgers and milk shakes.

No, I *didn't* want to contribute to the destruction of the environment.

Yes, I *did* want my life to be a statement of compassion. Which would be impossible as long as I was complicit in the torture and murder of billions of animals.

"That's it," I told Glen the moment the tape was over. "I ain't eating this shit anymore!"

Granted that's not the most articulate way to announce a major life decision, but it was how I felt then and it's how I still feel to this day:

I. Ain't. Eating. This. Shit. Anymore!

I hadn't woken up that morning planning on becoming a vegan, but from that moment on I was going to work at changing my life for the better. There was no turning back.

Before we go any further, however, I want to address a very simple but important question some of you might be asking: What exactly does *being a vegan* even mean?

The most basic definition of a vegan is someone who doesn't eat any meat, dairy, or fish. That means avoiding obvious products like hamburgers, chicken wings, pork chops, and scrambled eggs, as well as some that might not be so obvious as first. For instance, a plain slice of pizza isn't vegan, because cheese comes from cows (though you can get delicious vegan pizza—more on that later). Just as ice cream isn't vegan because it contains dairy. Or marshmallows aren't vegan because they contain gelatin, which is made out of the hooves and shins of horses.

This might sound like a New Age philosophy, but people have been warning against eating animals for thousands of years. The Lord Buddha said, "The eating of meat extinguishes the seed of great compassion." The Greek philosopher Plato was a vegetarian who noted that the more meat a society eats, the more doctors it needs. Leonardo da Vinci rejected eating meat, as did the great Russian novelist Leo Tolstoy, who wrote, "Flesh eating is simply immoral, as it involves the performance of an act, which is contrary to moral feeling: killing." Gandhi didn't eat meat either, telling his followers, "I do feel that spiritual progress does demand at some stage that we should cease to kill our fellow creatures for the satisfaction of our bodily wants."

The concept that a fully compassionate and healthy lifestyle required removing not only meat but also dairy from one's diet first gained traction in England shortly before World War II. At that time, 42 percent of Britain's cows had been found to be carrying tuberculosis. A group of concerned vegetarians decided to form an organization alerting people to the dangers of dairy. The group's founder, a woodcutter named Donald Watson, came up with the name the *Vegan Society*. "Vegan," he said, was meant to refer to both "the beginning and end of vegetarian."

Veganism picked up steam over the next few decades. Following the war, dairy production, as well as chicken, cow, and pig farms, became highly industrialized. Conditions became increasingly unsanitary and inhumane. There were more and more outbreaks of disease and mounting evidence that meat and dairy were bad for your health.

By the 1980s, groups like People for the Ethical Treatment of Animals (PETA) and the Animal Liberation Front had been formed to help promote a cruelty-free lifestyle. In 1988, *Diet for a New America* hit the shelves. In 1990, Robbins was joined by Lisa Bonet, Raul Julia, and River Phoenix on a special edition of *The Phil Donahue Show* about veganism that was watched by millions. The vegan lifestyle was here to stay.

Today, the vegan lifestyle is more mainstream than ever. Famous vegans include Bill Clinton, Ellen DeGeneres, Alicia Silverstone, Samuel L. Jackson, Miley Cyrus, Woody Harrelson, Mike Tyson, Erykah Badu, and André 3000 of OutKast. Not to mention vegetarians like

Deepak Chopra, Forest Whitaker, Prince, Angela Bassett, Omar Epps, and the author Jonathan Safran Foer. Many more celebrities, like Beyoncé, Jay Z, Jennifer Lopez, Venus Williams, and RZA from the Wu-Tang Clan have experimented with vegan diets in recent years. Oprah even had her entire staff (over three hundred people!) go on a weeklong vegan challenge.

Why are all these successful and famous people promoting what seems on the surface to be such a radical lifestyle change?

I believe it has to do with a dirty little secret about success and fame:

They don't necessarily make you happy.

Sure, playing with toys that accompany success and fame can make you happy for a minute. I won't lie, it feels great to drive a brand-new Rolls Royce off the lot. But after a few weeks of it, you realize that it's just a car. That's when you start asking yourself, "Now what?"

It's the same with new houses, exotic vacations, expensive clothes, even sex. After you experience enough of those things, you'll find yourself asking, "Now what?"

If you're being honest with yourself, the answer isn't "more of the same." That's because the truth is, the only things that are going to bring lasting happiness to your life are good health and knowledge of self, which lead to a compassionate relationship with the world.

That's it.

If your health and connection to yourself (as well as the larger world) are out of alignment, there aren't enough new cars, watches, or money in the world to make you happy.

I suspect most of the successful and famous people I just named experienced one of those "Now what?" moments, where they realized their toys weren't enough. Achievement wasn't enough. Fame wasn't enough.

If they wanted to find real happiness, they had to improve their health and their relationship with the world. And whether it was through research, the advice of a friend, or the example of someone they respected, they decided giving up animal products was the best way to do that.

What I'm asking you to do with this book is basically skip several steps in that process. Don't wait until you're having a "Now what?" moment, or even worse, a sobering talk with your doctor, to start that transformation. Start that process today.

Trust me, you won't be alone in making that move. When you go vegan, you will not be shutting yourself off from the world. Rather, you'll be joining a growing community of happy, successful, compassionate, and healthy people—a community that will welcome you with open arms.

It's also a community that grows stronger every year. In the last decade, searches for "vegan" on Google have doubled. Restaurant chains like Subway and Chipotle have introduced vegan options to their menus. Seemingly every month there's a new vegan restaurant opening or a new vegan product being added to supermarket shelves. The other day I was in New York and decided to pop in on a vegan street fair, but when I got there they were turning people away at the gates. Despite expecting thousands, the fair was already at capacity after just a couple of hours.

It's been amazing to watch this movement grow.

And now I want you to join me in it.

My argument is going to come down to three main points, the first of which is do it for health. As I'll detail, eating meat is directly linked to heart disease, the number one killer in America. It's also linked to cancer, our second-largest killer. Meat also increases your chances of developing deadly conditions like diabetes and Alzheimer's, which are the sixth and seventh leading killers in this country. No wonder studies have shown that you can add thirteen years to your life by giving up animal products. As someone on the other side of fifty, that's a very meaningful number.

Of course, giving up animal products isn't just about living longer; it's about getting the most out of your time here on earth too. When you go vegan you are likely going to lose weight (I dropped about twenty pounds). You're definitely going to feel better. Your energy level will increase and your recovery time from injuries will go down. Plus, when you become more mindful of what you put in your body every day, that mindfulness will seep into everything you do. Instead of sleepwalking through your life, you'll be more adept at living in the present moment. And the present, as I like to say, is the only place where good things can happen to you in life.

My second point will be that by giving up animal products, you won't only be potentially saving your own life. You'll help save Mother Earth too. Because, simply put, our appetite for animals is killing the planet.

I'll describe how the resources required to kill ten billion land animals a year in America alone is destroying our fields, polluting our air, and poisoning our waters. Few realize this, but livestock production contributes more to global warming than cars, planes, and trains *combined*. You can consider yourself an "environmentalist" because you drive a Prius, recycle your plastics, and take shorter showers. But at the end of the day you're just playing with yourself when you do that. Sorry, but none of those practices would help the environment as much as simply giving up animal products.

The final argument I'll present for eating a plant-based diet will center on compassion. The terror and pain we inflict on the billions of animals that are born into suffering every year is the worst karmic disaster in the history of the world. Subconsciously we all know the conditions these animals face are bad, but when you clean off your lenses and take a clear look at the facts, you will see just how revolting the situation truly is.

What I'm going to tell you about factory farming will probably gross you out. But if you eat meat, then you need to read it. You can't avoid the truth about products you are putting into your body *every single day*. Literally, nothing could affect you more directly. You owe it to yourself to confront this information head-on.

If you think I'm being judgmental toward meat eaters, I promise I'm not here to make anyone feel bad about their choices. How could I? Whatever you've put in your body, trust me, I've put worse in mine. That didn't make me a bad person then, just as it doesn't make you a bad person now.

Instead of making you feel defensive, I simply want this book to help you look at your choices differently. I want these words to cut through the noise that's been distracting you.

I can't blame you for being distracted. From childhood, you have been subjected to a billion-dollar propaganda campaign designed to distract you from the effect animal products are having on your body, your karma, and the earth. From the packaging your chicken breasts are wrapped in to the commercials you've seen on TV, you've been lied to every step of the way. I can't fault anyone for falling victim to those lies.

I do, however, firmly believe in this simple maxim:

People who *know* better *do* better.

If you've even made it this far into the introduction, then you *do* want to do better. You do want to know what's going on with the food you put in your body. You *do* want to know how you can feel healthier and more alive. You *do* want to know how you can strengthen your connection to the planet.

You're someone who asks questions and isn't comfortable blindly following the pack. It wasn't for a lack of effort, but the meat and dairy industries haven't been able to completely desensitize you to the suffering that's out there.

So no matter which boxes you check when you're asked to describe yourself—"vegan," "vegetarian," "black," "Christian," "woman," "carnivore," "yogi," "liberal," "conservative," "gay," "straight," or whatever— there's a part of you that does want to explore a better route through life.

Which is why I'm confident that when you do know the facts, switching to a plant-based diet will be an easy choice for you to make.

Easy is a word that few people associate with giving up food they've been eating their entire lives. Even if you decide you *want* to switch after reading this book, you might have real concerns about whether you *can* do it.

I want to get those concerns out of the way first, which is why I'm going to start off the book by debunking some of the most common misconceptions about being a vegan:

- Eating meat is a fundamental part of your cultural tradition.
- There's something weird or antisocial about giving up meat.
- Only rich people can afford to go vegan.
- You need to be an animal lover to be committed to a vegan lifestyle.
- You're no good at dieting.

In short, that it's just too hard.

Once those misconceptions are cleared up and I've shared all the information on why you should give up animal products, then I'm going to teach you how to do it. I'm going to show you which items need to be banished from your kitchen and which ones you need to start stocking up on. I'm going to tell you which products to start looking for at the supermarket and which ones to avoid. As well as what to order when you go out to eat with your meat-eating friends. I'm also going to share a list of websites for you to visit to help you find vegan restaurants and markets in your area as well as cookbooks that can help you start preparing delicious vegan meals on your own.

Thank you in advance for allowing me to get you started on this journey. There might be a few bumps in the road. A few frustrating moments where you wonder if you've made the right choice. Don't let those moments of doubt trip you up, or even worse, make you turn around.

As long as you stay on this path, you'll realize you truly can do anything. You can save money. You can look better. You can have more energy. You can lose weight. You can save the animals. You can save the world.

THE MISCONCEPTIONS

I LOVE MEAT TOO MUCH TO GIVE IT UP

> *"I thought, like with most diets, I would feel deprived and hate food, that I would miss out on restaurants and celebrations, that I would get headaches and be irritable, etc. I was wrong about all of that. It took a few days to adjust, but what I discovered was increased energy, better sleep, weight loss, improved digestion, clarity, and an incredible positive feeling for my actions and the effect it would have on those around me and on the environment. I couldn't believe how much of our health we control with food."* —BEYONCÉ ON HER PLANT-BASED DIET

For many people, the biggest perceived barrier to becoming a vegan is simply how much they love eating meat. "Russell, you don't get it," they'll tell me. "Ribs taste soooo good. We have a special relationship. How could I give them up?"

There's almost a perception that if you don't eat meat, you must have *never* eaten meat. Because if you had, then you wouldn't even *dream* of suggesting that someone else give it up.

But I have.

And I am.

Trust me, I ate meat with the best of them. I often joke that I would have eaten an elephant's ass if someone had put it on a plate in front of me, but I'm not really kidding. I would've chewed it up and probably asked for seconds.

My favorite dish was my mother's spaghetti with peppers and sausage. She used to make it with these giant sausages she'd get from a butcher on Hollis Avenue, the main drag in Hollis, Queens, where we lived. Nothing was better than coming in from a day of running around the streets and see her in the kitchen cooking a big pot of it.

My mother also made a delicious oxtail stew. She'd prepare it with potatoes and carrots and let it cook for a long time, so the beef would just be falling off the bone by the time it was done.

My father could cook too; his signature dish was pig's feet with potato salad and collard greens. His people were from down South and he would take pride in reminding us that pig's feet were what "real niggers" ate. Not that bougie stuff that folks up North tried to pass off as "soul food."

I used to start my day off with meat. If I came downstairs in the morning and saw that my mother hadn't cooked a plate of bacon and eggs, then I'd head down to Hollis Avenue and grab a sausage sandwich with jelly. Even after I'd launched Def Jam Records and had enough money to order anything I wanted for breakfast, I'd still send an intern out every morning to grab me a sausage sandwich with jelly.

When I was out on the road with rappers like Kurtis Blow, Run-D.M.C., The Beastie Boys, and LL Cool J, our go-to meal was hamburgers. My personal favorites were Burger King and Jack in the Box, though some of the guys used to prefer McDonald's. And for the record it was Glen—yes, *that* Glen—who first put the Beasties on to Fatburger, the Los Angeles chain. That's significant for two reasons: First, it shows that even a hard-core vegan like Glen used to love hamburgers. Second, the Beasties actually helped popularize Fatburger nationally in their song "The New Style" when they rhymed: "I chill at White Castle 'cause it's the best / but I'm fly at Fatburger when I'm way out west."

If we weren't eating burgers, we were probably digging into a big bucket of fried chicken. Kentucky Fried Chicken was always popular, but my personal favorite was Bojangles's fried chicken with Delta sauce and dirty rice. I used to get excited when I'd see cities like Atlanta or Savannah on our tour itinerary because I knew I'd get a chance to have some of that Bojangles's.

Once I started making some real money, I tried to expand my tastes a bit. Instead of White Castle or KFC, I liked to go out and get sushi or paella, which in the 1980s most folks in hip-hop weren't up on yet. I'd take a bunch of rappers out to dinner, and they'd want lobster and steak, but I'd insist on going to an Indian place instead and getting the chicken masala.

My mother never made chitlins when I was growing up, but I started ordering them whenever I went to a soul food place in Manhattan's West Village called the Pink Tea Cup. I used to sit there at a table filled with models and record executives and order *chitlins*. That never used to go over too well.

By now you should be getting the point: I used to enjoy eating meat. From my mother's spaghetti and sausage to a Burger King Whopper to the chitlins at the Pink Tea Cup, I loved how all those dishes tasted.

But here's the thing—*I don't miss them.*

When you give up animal products, it's not like you're also giving up delicious meals. Instead you just start eating different *kinds* of delicious meals. I'm still going out for Indian food, it's just that now I'm getting the kaali dal (black lentils) instead of the chicken masala. When I get Thai food, I'm getting the vegetable pad thai with a side of coconut curry instead of the chicken pad thai. Those dishes might not contain animal products, but they're still delicious.

If you're incredulous that I could find lentils as delicious as a lamb chop or tofu as tasty as a tuna steak, understand this: My taste buds have changed since I stopped eating animal products.

Almost every vegan I know has had a similar experience. Here's why: Most meat dishes—especially processed fast foods—contain lots of salt, fat, and sugar. Heavy flavors that dull your taste buds over time. It's why really greasy pork chops or super salty sausages *seem* to taste so good. Your taste buds have become so dulled that unless there's a ton of salt and fat in a dish, you're not going to taste anything.

But after just a few weeks of not eating animal products—and all the salt, fat, and sugar that usually accompany it—your taste buds are going to be reborn. You're going to start picking up on all the subtle but powerful flavors that are used in vegetarian dishes like curry, tahini, moles, and pestos. You're going to savor the aroma of slow-cooked onions and garlic, of braised potatoes and turnips, of potatoes roasted with rosemary. You're going to start to appreciate the texture in quinoa (a grain that's a great addition to a vegan diet), mushrooms, beans, as well as the crispness of fresh vegetables like raw peppers and cucumbers.

If you do go back to animal products, they probably won't taste as good as you remember them. You might say "BS," but if you've ever quit smoking cigarettes, you know how disgusting it can be to be around someone who's smoking, let alone smoking yourself. You might almost throw up at the thought of it. It's not much different with food. A lot of folks report that if they try meat after going without it for a while, it tastes way too greasy to them. Just as many say that if they go back to cheese, it tastes too oily and salty.

> "Getting rid of the dairy was great, getting rid of the meat—I just don't miss it."
> —Bill Clinton

The idea that our taste buds can change shouldn't be hard to accept. After all, don't most of our tastes change? When I was a kid, you couldn't have convinced me that there was anything greater than a Mighty Mouse cartoon. And in that moment, there wasn't. But eventually my taste in TV changed. When I was a teenager, I listened to a lot of R&B. When I was in college, I heard hip-hop and fell in love with that. My taste in music evolved. When I was fifteen I thought there weren't any clothes flyer than mock turtlenecks and AJ Lester slacks. Today I prefer argyle vests and jeans. My tastes have changed in a lot of areas as I've grown. My taste buds are no different.

A yoga teacher once told me: "A yogi steadily loses the taste for things that don't taste good," and I've found that to be true. We lose our desires for many things that aren't good for us: drugs, booze, illicit sex, and drama. But I think it's especially true of our taste for meat.

I'd always assumed I couldn't live without animal products, but both my body and my spirit were more than happy to let them go. Physically, I started feeling the difference in just a few weeks. I had more energy and slept better at night. My mind became clearer and my focus grew stronger. My taste buds stopped craving those heavy, greasy flavors and started appreciating lighter and more diverse seasonings.

> "The longer we eat healthier foods, the better they taste."
> —Dr. Michael Greger, Humane Society

Most important, I felt better about my relationship with the world. It's a relief to disconnect yourself from a system that's causing harm and suffering. When you cleanse yourself of that negativity, it brightens your whole outlook.

Even though I grew up in a world where every "good" meal had to include meat, where a glass of milk was the symbol of health, I was able to grow out of that mentality.

My yoga teacher was right: I *had* lost my appetite for something that wasn't good for me anymore. And you will too.

PEOPLE HAVE ALWAYS EATEN MEAT; IT'S JUST NATURAL

"Although we think we are, and we act as if we are, human beings are not natural carnivores. When we kill animals to eat them, they end up killing us, because their flesh, which contains cholesterol and saturated fat, was never intended for human beings, who are natural herbivores."

—DR. WILLIAM C. ROBERTS,

AMERICAN JOURNAL OF CARDIOLOGY

A lot of folks out there want to believe that humans were *meant* to be carnivores, or animals that eat meat. But vegans believe, and science backs us up, that while humans have eaten meat throughout history, we are naturally better suited to a herbivorous, or vegetarian, diet. If you look at carnivorous animals like lions or tigers, they all have long, curved fangs and claws, as well as short digestive tracts. Their fangs and claws allow them to rip and tear the meat they eat, and their short digestive tracts process the meat before it has time to rot.

Humans, on the other hand, have flat, flexible nails, and our so-called canine teeth are minuscule compared to carnivores'. Human teeth are better suited to biting into vegetables, fruits, and grains than tearing through tough hides.

This is why Neal Barnard, president of the Physicians Committee for Responsible Medicine, writes in his book *The Power of Your Plate*, "Early humans had diets very much like other great apes, which is to say a largely plant-based diet, drawing on foods we can pick with our hands.

Research suggests that meat-eating probably began by scavenging—eating the leftovers that carnivores had left behind. However, our bodies have never adapted to it. To this day, meat-eaters have a higher incidence of heart disease, cancer, diabetes, and other problems."

"Well," you might be saying, "even if early man wasn't designed to eat meat specifically, that's what my relatives were still doing for all these years." But even that's only partially true. Yes, some humans have always eaten meat. But not in every culture. And certainly not on every level of society. No matter where your ancestors are from—West Africa, Ireland, China, Mexico, or Italy—chances are, they were not the big meat eaters that you might assume they were.

Let's say you're Irish American. For St. Patrick's Day you might serve corned beef and cabbage. Because what's more Irish than corned beef and cabbage? Well, it turns out almost *everything*. That's because while corned beef might have become popular with your fellow Irish Americans, none of your ancestors back in Ireland actually ate it.

That's right, corned beef and cabbage didn't become popular as a dish until Irish immigrants came to America and had access to affordable beef. Back in Ireland, their diet consisted almost exclusively of potatoes, cabbage, leeks, and carrots. Exactly the kind of low-fat, plant-based diet I'm going to promote in this book.

What they *weren't* eating was meat. The vast majority of Irish were dirt-poor peasants who lived on the estates of rich British landowners. If there was any meat to be had, the British landowners were getting it, not your Irish relatives. Remember, a million people died in the Irish *Potato* Famine, not the Irish Beef Famine.

The truth is, most Irish immigrants had never even *tasted* beef before they got to the United States. There are records of newly arrived Irish immigrants writing back to their relatives, "You won't believe it, but people get to eat meat over here!" Forget about the streets paved with gold—the Irish immigrants were excited that they could eat beef and pork for the first time.

It's a similar story around the world. Today, you might go into a Chinese restaurant and order a General Tso's chicken, but that's not representative of traditional Chinese food. Until very recently, when China began to copy a Western diet, most people in China didn't eat much meat. Instead, they ate a lot of soybeans, grains, and vegetables. When there was meat in a dish, it was only in small amounts and generally used as seasoning. Maybe a little ground pork or dried fish sprinkled over rice. But big chunks of chicken like you get in General Tso's? Or thick hunks of meat like you get in your beef and broccoli? You wouldn't find that in a traditional Chinese meal.

I don't think anyone holds on to the myth that meat is somehow a fundamental part of their heritage more closely than African Americans. So let's take a closer look at the history of meat and African Americans and dispel this fairy tale once and for all.

If you're African American, your ancestors likely came from West Africa, a region that today comprises countries like Ghana, Benin, Senegal, and Sierra Leone. Do you know what makes up the traditional diets in those countries? Not meat. It's yams, cassava, melons, bananas, okra, sweet potato, and porridge. Again, the same kind of plant-based diet I'm going to encourage you to eat in this book.

If they came from a coastal region, maybe they ate a little salted fish from time to time. But meat? Your West African ancestors ate meat only at big occasions, like a wedding or a funeral. Even then, as in China, it would mainly only be used for flavoring. Your African ancestors were not chowing down on a big plate of ribs or eating two dozen chicken wings in a sitting. Unless they were part of a wealthy king or chief's family, there was just no way they could afford that.

Ham hocks? Ribs? Pig's feet? Chitlins? Those are not African dishes. Those are *slave* dishes. Never forget that! They were introduced into our ancestors' diets only once they were put in chains and brought over to plantations in the Caribbean and North America. Do you know why okra and red beans, which are originally from West Africa, became popular in the South? Because when the first slaves got here, they wouldn't eat the heavily salted pork the plantation owners were trying to feed them. Since those slave owners wanted to protect their investment, they had their ships bring okra and red bean seeds back from West Africa. Otherwise their slaves wouldn't eat.

Hundreds of years later, we've forgotten that our ancestors largely lived on a plant-based diet. We've gotten so conditioned to cheap meat that today we cling to it as a fundamental part of our culture. Worse, we get suspicious, even insulted, when someone suggests giving it up.

I see this misplaced outrage toward vegans from African Americans on Twitter all the time. One person tweeted, "My uncle brought a vegan date to Thanksgiving dinner & she asked were the greens cooked in pork. Grandma had to be restrained." I saw another guy post, "Me & shawty just had a convo on why she's a vegan. She better be glad I like her enough to keep her around. What black folk don't eat chicken?"

Those tweets were obviously meant to be funny, but as the saying goes, all good comedy is based in truth. I addressed this mind-set in my last book, *Success Through Stillness*, when I wrote, "Growing up, it was almost as if eating 'comfort food' was the most accessible way of dealing with the stresses, disappointments, and injustices that seemed to be inherent to the African American experience. If you questioned your plate of ham hocks, black-eyed peas, and corn bread, it was almost like you were questioning your blackness."

We've got to move past that mentality and confront the damage animal products wreak on our community. Largely because of its meat-based diet, the African American community is disproportionately affected by diseases like high blood pressure, high cholesterol, strokes, and diabetes. For instance, according to the U.S. Department of Health and Human Services (DHHS), African Americans are 40 percent more likely to develop high blood pressure than other ethnic groups. It's especially bad for African American women, who the DHHS estimates are 30 percent more likely to die from heart disease than white men.

"The real hallmark of being human isn't our taste for meat but our ability to adapt to many habitats—and to be able to combine many different foods to create many healthy diets. Unfortunately the modern Western diet does not appear to be one of them."

—*National Geographic,* "The Evolution of Diet"

I can quote you statistics all day, but if you're African American you probably have experienced this firsthand already. How many people in your family have been affected or, even worse, killed by one of these diseases? How many have passed away from heart disease? How many are laid up in a home after suffering a stroke? Or lost a limb to diabetes? There have certainly been too many in mine.

What's so heartbreaking is those are all largely *preventable* diseases. Which could be avoided by taking animal products out of our diets. We're quick to talk shit on Twitter about someone who won't eat meat at a cookout, yet we're quiet as mice when the fast-food chains push low-quality meat in every urban area. Just as we don't have much to say when the milk marketers create ads specifically targeting African Americans and Hispanics. We've got to wake up to what's happening.

I remember hearing Bob Law (one of the first stars of African American talk radio) share a very insightful observation about the relationship between black folks and meat. I'm paraphrasing, but it was something to the effect of, "The brilliance of black folk is not that they can make chitlins so good, it's that they can make chitlins *so good*."

In other words, how incredible was it that as a people we were given crap—chitlins were literally the shit-stained intestines from pigs that slave owners refused to eat—but still managed to turn it into a delicacy? Bob was saying, Let's celebrate how adaptable and inventive African Americans have been in the face of so many hardships and crises: that we could take scraps and turn them into something that, over four hundred years later, someone like me would pay top dollar for at the Pink Tea Cup.

What I'm arguing is that we need to take that same brilliance and ingenuity and apply it to a *new* crisis we're facing. Four hundred years ago, we didn't have any choices. It was either eat the crap thrown in front of us or starve. Today, we have an unbelievable amount of options when it comes to what we put in our bodies. To keep making the same choices we've always made, in the face of so much suffering and death, is insane.

As black folks we protest—as we should—an education system that leaves too many of our young people without the skills they need to succeed in the workforce. We protest a lending system that simultaneously discriminates against and preys on us. We protest a prison system that disproportionally throws our young men in jail and profits off of unfair drug laws. And we protest—very loudly—a system that allows police officers to profile and often kill our young people without any repercussions.

Yet when it comes to a diet that is in large part responsible for the death of more than a hundred thousand African Americans each year, again we barely make a peep. In fact, not only don't we speak out against it, we celebrate it!

I'm going to be very real here: As terrible as it is to have a relative or friend thrown in jail over some BS weed charge or to have them beaten up by a dirty cop, odds are the biggest threat looming over your family and friends is their diets.

You might not have had a choice about what sort of school you went to as a kid or how a police officer reacts to your skin color when he pulls you over. Those things are often out of your hands. But you do have a say about what you put in your body every day—that choice is literally *in your hands*.

I also hear some people say, "Sorry, I'm addicted to chicken; I just can't give it up." Sorry, but that's BS. I've been addicted to things before (I'll discuss this more in the "How to Do It" chapter), but despite how much of it I consumed, meat was never one of them. *Nobody* is addicted to meat. A drug addict has to get sent off to rehab, or more likely, locked in a cage before he can make a change. Not you. Your cage is only mental. All you have to do is make that compassionate choice to open up the door and set yourself free.

I've been addressing the situation in the African American community, but it holds true for everyone reading this book. Each and every one of us can make the choice to stop consuming animal products and switch over to a plant-based diet. Rich, poor, middle class—it doesn't matter. *Everyone* can afford to go vegan. What you can't afford is *not* to.

In fact, let's tackle the misconception that you have to be rich to enjoy a vegan lifestyle next.

> "Consider your health: Fresh organic fruits and vegetables may cost more than some junk foods, but isn't your health worth the extra couple of bucks? [. . .] Given the health benefits of a vegan diet, you'll likely save hundreds or thousands of dollars on health care, which will more than make up for the extra cost of soy milk."
>
> —PETA

ONLY RICH PEOPLE CAN AFFORD TO GO VEGAN

Maybe I'm a little more sensitive because I'm rich myself, but I feel like I encounter the perception that "only rich people can afford to go vegan" quite a bit. Especially when Beyoncé and Jay Z decided to go on a twenty-two-day vegan challenge in 2014.

In announcing his decision, Jay wrote that he was motivated to give up meat and switch to a plant-based diet after an unnamed friend urged him to experience "optimum wellness through conscious nutrition."

A lot of people thought *I* was that friend, but I can't take the credit. Bey and Jay were actually motivated by the nutritionist Marco Borges, who also helped J. Lo give up animal products. I was, of course, super supportive of the challenge and tweeted, "Welcome to the club, Jay and Bey!" Besides being happy for them personally, I was also excited that it would motivate their fans to try a plant-based diet too.

> "It just feels right!"
> —Jay Z on adopting a plant-based diet

Their challenge certainly achieved that: Bey and Borges recently launched a vegan meal-delivery service for all the fans who've made the switch, as well as collaborating on a best-selling cookbook. But when they made their initial announcement, and when Beyoncé later famously promoted her diet on *Good Morning America*, there was backlash on Twitter from fans complaining they couldn't follow Jay and Bey's lead without also having their kind of money:

"It's easy for jay z and bey to go vegan. they have caterers. ive always wanted to try and go vegan, but i never had the help or money"

"Beyoncé is rich. Filthy. She can afford 2make her vegan taste like steak & chicken. OUR vegan will taste like pencil shavings"

"If I had the money to pay a service for that, I'd do it."

I understand those concerns, but money isn't nearly the barrier some make it out to be. Look, is it easier to switch up your diet if you're rich? I'd be lying if I tried to tell you otherwise. Just as I'd be lying if I tried to tell you sending your kids to a good school or going on a nice vacation isn't also easier if you're rich.

But if you're not rich, does that mean you're not going to try to get your kid into the best school or stop going on family trips? Of course not. You're still going to put in the work and do the best you can for yourself and your family. Your approach shouldn't be any different with your diet.

My resources have allowed me to hire great chefs who cook delicious meals for me. I also have the option of eating out at vegan restaurants whenever I don't feel like cooking, which I'll admit is too often.

But even if you don't have those same kinds of resources, I want to convince you that you still don't need to be rich to switch to a plant-based diet. It's a change you can make without too much stress to your lifestyle or your pocketbook. And the best way to convince you is to look at the numbers.

Let's start with your grocery bills. If you were to itemize all the money you spend on food each month, you'd probably find meat and dairy accounts for somewhere between 10 and 20 percent of your budget.

If you were to cut out all those hamburger patties, chicken breasts, and pork loins and replace them with vegetables, grains, and fruits, you'd save a lot of money. To put it in perspective, a pound of organic lentils costs around $2. In 2014, a pound of regular beef costs close to $4. A pound of organic beef (without hormones and antibiotics) runs close to $10.

According to *Forbes*, Americans spend $142 billion annually on beef, chicken, pork, turkey, and lamb.

Instead of making meat loaf, you could make a delicious lentil loaf with carrots and celery. Instead of hamburger, you could cook vegetarian chili. If you ended up replacing all the meat you cooked with vegetables and other plant-based foods, how much do you think you'd save over the course of a year? Studies have shown close to $4,000. Extended to a family of four, you could save roughly $16,000 a year by giving up meat.

That's a significant number. In fact, I can't think of a lot of other lifestyle changes your family could make that would save you sixteen grand per year. Maybe tell your kids they can't get braces. Maybe cancel your summer vacation. Or stop heating your house in the winter. Doesn't simply eating a healthier diet sound like a better alternative to those sorts of changes?

Ordering vegan when you eat out isn't going to be that much more expensive either. If you eat a lot of fast food in order to save money, that doesn't have to change. I still go to Taco Bell, where I get the bean burrito. I just ask them to replace the cheese with guacamole. There's no extra charge, and they're always happy to do it.

If you like Burger King, get the BK Veggie Whopper, which costs the same as the regular Whopper. Or if you love Chipotle, you can get sofritas, which are braised organic tofu, in your burrito, bowl, or salad. It's actually cheaper than the meat options. I would encourage you to stay away from fast food as much as possible because it's highly processed, but if that's what fits your budget now, you can still do it without eating animal products.

It's going to be a similar story if you want to eat at more upscale restaurants. In L.A., my favorite vegan spot is Crossroads in Hollywood, which is very popular with the city's rich and famous.

The legendary actor James Caan is there so much I joke he might as well be one of the bar stools. Not long ago, my assistant Simone was at Crossroads getting dinner when Jay Z, Beyoncé, Warren Beatty, and Bill Clinton all came in to eat at the same time. Simone told me before she realized President Clinton was there, she thought the Secret Service were there for Jay and Beyoncé!

But even a vegan restaurant so hip that Jay, Beyoncé, and Bill Clinton can literally bump into each other there still isn't that expensive. When I go to Crossroads, I usually order the wood-fired "meaty" lasagna. It's delicious and it costs $16. Definitely not cheap, but a *lot less* than I would be paying for a meat entrée at a fancy French restaurant or a sushi platter at an upscale Japanese place.

In fact, the "meaty" lasagna at ultra-upscale Crossroads isn't that much more expensive than the lasagna classico at the Olive Garden, which costs $13.29. Proof you don't really need to have Beyoncé's and Jay Z's kind of money to afford a great plant-based dinner.

Sure, there are going to be moments where it's going to cost you more to eat vegan. You might have to pick a salad that's more expensive than a Big Mac. Or get a plate of pasta instead of a slice of pizza. But remember, you're saving four grand a year right off the top by eliminating meat from your grocery bill. So you're going to have some extra money in your pocket to make up the difference.

Let me also say something about all those cheap burgers and chicken wings that might be helping you get by on a limited budget: They shouldn't be so cheap.

The reason you're able to get a Big Mac for $5 or six chicken wings and pork fried rice at a Chinese takeout place for only $3.99 is because our government has spent a ton of money keeping meat prices artificially low.

According to PETA, our government provides the meat and dairy industries with $38 *billion* in subsidies every single year. By comparison, they give the fruit and vegetable industries only $17 million a year, just 0.04 percent of what they earmark for animal products.

In his book *Meatonomic$*, David Robinson Simon estimates that the meat and dairy industries end up costing our economy a staggering $414 billion a year in "hidden costs." That figure reflects the subsidies the meat and dairy industries receive from our government, the environmental damage they cause, and the health-care costs of people who become sick from their products. Simon says that if you factored in all those costs, the "real" price of a Big Mac should actually be closer to $13.

Or consider the artificial pricing in the poultry industry. Back in

1935, the retail price for a pound of chicken (adjusted for inflation) was $5.07. Today, that same pound of chicken costs you about $1.60. That might not seem like a big deal, but consider this: The average price (again adjusted) for a new car in 1935 was $11,200. Today it's $32,000. The cost of a new home in 1935 was $59,400. Today, it's around $275,000. In 1935, a gallon of gas would have cost you $1.72. Today, it might run you $3 or $4.

In almost every other category, items cost much more today than they did in 1935. Chicken actually costs *less*. This is because our government is giving massive subsidies to the poultry industry. Those subsidies are often indirect and come in the form of the government buying "unwanted" chicken directly from the producers. It's essentially corporate welfare. According to the *Wall Street Journal*, in 2011 alone our government spent $186 million purchasing chicken meat that otherwise wouldn't have been sold. A Tufts University report claims that the poultry industry as a whole saved over *$11 billion* in costs between 1997 and 2005 on taxpayer-funded subsidies of the corn and soybeans many poultry producers use for chicken feed.

Whether chicken, pork, beef, or turkey, all this cheap meat isn't a smart choice for our country. Especially when we have so many other sectors—education and health care being foremost—that need government subsidies way more than the Purdue family does.

We talk about a housing bubble, or a tech bubble, or the college loan bubble, but to me the meat and dairy bubble is the most serious of them all. We've got a whole nation of people programmed to think that it's somehow their right to have access to cheap meat all the time.

Let's rethink how we spend our money on food. Both collectively and individually. Yes, you might have to pay a little bit out of pocket when you first give up animal products. But then consider where you'll really be saving by giving up animal products: your health-care costs. It sounds almost silly to say, but having heart disease is *expensive*. Living with diabetes is expensive. Open-heart surgery is expensive. As is chemotherapy.

I'm talking only about the cost of missing work, the cost of living on prescription pills, the costs of constant hospital visits. To say nothing of the emotional tax of fighting a disease.

When you factor in all those costs, there's no way you can look at switching to a plant-based diet and say, "I can't afford to do this." You should say, "I can't afford *not* to do this."

Please make spending money on healthful food your top priority. There's no better investment than a diet built on organic vegetables and fruit. If you're reading this book, I'm guessing you think I know what I'm talking about—at least a little bit—when it comes to business. You'd probably listen if I told you to invest in a new media company. Or a certain stock. Or a certain type of bond. I have a pretty strong track record with that sort of stuff. So I hope you'll hear me very clearly when I say spending money on eating right is the *single* best investment you could possibly make with your money.

There's no doubt that as a society, one of our greatest challenges moving forward is to find a way to bring affordable organic fruits and vegetables to poorer communities, especially in urban areas. For most of human history, meat has been expensive and veggies were cheap and plentiful. In America today, we've turned that upside down.

Vegetables and fruits need to be both available and more affordable in the corner stores and bodegas as well as in school lunchrooms and vending machines. We need to make it just as easy for a single mother to pick up a spicy lentil and onion wrap on her way home as a Quarter Pounder with fries. And for a kid leaving school to have access to a great-tasting quinoa salad just as easily as he would a slice of pizza. Personally, I'm committed to making what I just described a reality. It's one of the main reasons I'm writing this book.

But until we collectively make that shift, I'm encouraging you to make it on your own first. It will be a heroic stance for you to take. You're going to be removing yourself from an exploitive and harmful system and showing your family and friends a smarter and healthier way to live through your actions. Instead of being part of the problem, you're going to be part of the solution.

That's what being a hero is all about.

PEOPLE WILL THINK I'M WEIRD

> *"Caring about what you eat and trying to make it tasty and educate the public is not some kind of fringe activity of tree huggers but a matter of fundamental survival and continued vitality of our society starting right here."*
>
> —STEVE WYNN, CASINO MOGUL, AT THE OPENING
> OF HIS RESTAURANT VIVA LAS VEGAN

I'll be honest: Even though I'm going to call you a hero for giving up animal products, not everyone else will.

They might call you weird. Or strange. Or even a freak.

Sadly, those perceptions are a major roadblock for many people thinking about starting this journey. Even folks who are normally progressive thinkers or consider themselves their "own man" or an "independent woman" still feel more comfortable running with the pack when it comes to the food they eat. Even when the pack is about to take them over the edge of a cliff.

Not me, though. I embrace being thought of as "weird" or "different." I won't skip a beat if someone makes a little comment about me serving vegan food at one of my parties or gives me a weird look if I ask a waiter about the animal-free options on a menu. I see those moments as a chance to create dialogue and open someone's mind up to possibilities they might not have considered before.

Plenty of people thought I was weird back in the '70s when I kept talking about how great these guys sound rapping on a microphone. Just as, later, plenty of people thought I was a little nuts when I said hip-hop could support its own fashion line. Or when I put spoken-word poetry on Broadway. Or had black comics like Kevin Hart and Bernie Mac cussin' on HBO. Whenever I'm going against the grain, I feel like I'm moving in the right direction.

You might not have the same mentality. Even though I know you're a free thinker just by the fact that you're taking the time to read this, it could take a while to locate the faith that you're doing the right thing. So let's address the reality that a lot of people, even those closest to you, might judge you negatively for giving up animal products.

The great irony is that one of the first things you'll be judged on is the perception that vegans are—you guessed it—judgmental. You'll hear complaints that vegans try to push their beliefs on everyone else. That they unfairly attack people who eat meat. That they're aloof.

Insufferable. As a friend of mine put it, "You vegans have this air of superiority about you. Like you're better than everyone else."

Don't let that sort of talk dissuade you. I hang out with vegans all the time, and I can say that as a community, they're actually some of the most open-minded, progressive, and *nonjudgmental* people I know. They're certainly in my experience less likely to be racist, homophobic, or misogynist. The types of judgments that *can* actually hurt people.

Now, are there some insufferable vegans out there?

Sure.

But guess what? They're probably a pain in the ass about most things, not just what they do or don't eat. I have a vegan friend who's got a stick up his butt about music. About fashion. And politics. He was pejorative way before he'd ever even heard the word *vegan*. It's not like the second he stopped eating meat he suddenly thought he knew better than everyone else. I love the guy, but he *always* thought he was making better choices than everyone else! His diet had nothing to do with it.

Instead of getting turned off by the idea of joining a group of elitist food snobs, it's more helpful to ask yourself, "Why do people feel so threatened by vegans? Why does the idea of giving up meat and dairy trigger a negative response?" Why would people who would normally be your biggest supporters be against a change that's going to improve your health and happiness?

One answer is that they've been manipulated into feeling that way. The meat and dairy industries spend over *$10 billion a year* in advertising (the fast-food industry alone spends $4 billion) to reinforce the perception that consuming their products is normal and that anyone who doesn't isn't.

That money is spent on campaigns like "Beef: It's What's for Dinner," "Milk: It Does a Body Good," and the ubiquitous "Got Milk?" featuring smiling athletes and celebrities wearing milk mustaches. Never mind that milk doesn't actually "do your body good," unless you happen to be a baby cow. Never mind that consuming dairy is more likely to slow you down than give you any extra strength. Never mind that fifty million Americans are lactose intolerant, including an estimated 70 percent of African Americans and 80 percent of Asian Americans and Jews. These campaigns have created the perception that meat and dairy are synonymous with health and vitality. When, in fact, nothing could be further from the truth.

Suppose we let drug dealers run similar campaigns. Maybe "Crack: Need a Little Lift?" Or "Heroin: Nod If You Love It!" I'm not sure they would be any more ludicrous than the falsehoods that the meat and dairy industries are putting out there. Or that results would be much worse for the American public.

What's most disturbing is the role our government plays in funding and spreading this misinformation. Every year, the U.S. Department of Agriculture (USDA) sets aside roughly $550 million that goes directly to organizations like the U.S. Cattlemen's Association or the National Pork Producers Council for ad campaigns. Our government's top priority should be protecting its citizens, but it is pushing poison on them instead. This is why I support movements like Occupy Wall Street and Black Lives Matter. When your government doesn't put the best interests of its citizens first, you have to say something about it.

Our government's twisted priorities are evidenced most clearly when the USDA promotes the Standard American Diet (SAD). We all grew up seeing that SAD food pyramid on our classroom walls and in pamphlets. It taught generations of Americans that meat and dairy should be an essential part of their diets.

In truth, that food pyramid was created by businesspeople as much as by doctors or nutritionists. Businesspeople who are happy to push death if it means more money. Just like their buddies in the tobacco industry and prison industrial complex. Our government is pay for play, and these businesspeople are just going to keep on playing—with our lives—until we let them know we've had enough and stop buying their products.

> "Almost any diet that takes us away from the Standard American Diet is an improvement."
> —Mark Bittman

That can be challenging, because they also try to shut down anyone who speaks out against what they're up to. Remember when Oprah Winfrey said she wasn't going to eat any more hamburgers during an outbreak of mad cow disease? The beef industry poured all its resources into coming after her. They called her a liar. They took her to court and sued her for $10 million. Of course Oprah stood up to their tactics and refused to be silenced. After a jury found in her favor, she told the press, "I'm still off hamburgers." But if they came after someone as beloved and respected as Oprah, imagine how hard they must come after people who don't have Oprah's platform or resources.

It's impossible to overstate just how deeply the meat and dairy industries have manipulated Americans' attitudes toward what we eat. Try going on Twitter or Facebook and posting something about not eating animal products. You might only be talking about your own choices, but you can expect a bunch of angry meat eaters to show up in your timeline. If you're at a party and ask about the vegetarian options, don't be shocked if someone makes a snide little comment about people who don't eat meat. People have been programmed to think you're doing something wrong.

Falling prey to propaganda is only part of it, though. My experience has made me believe that when people criticize vegans, they're often projecting their own insecurity about their own diet. If someone feels the need to attack your decision *not* to eat animals, that person has to be in some sort of pain themselves. There's simply no other rational explanation as to why *they'd* become outraged by *your* food choices. *Especially* healthy ones.

Whether it's a physical or physiological pain can be hard to tell, but only someone uncomfortable with their own situation would try to make you feel that way about yours. This is why when someone has a beef (pun intended) with my healthy food choices, I always try to remember the maxim "Hurt people hurt people."

Compassion is why so many of us become vegan in the first place, but it can't just be extended to animals. We also have to be compassionate toward our critics, even if their criticism isn't warranted.

It can be tough when those critics might be your partners, spouses, and parents. Your husband might complain, "If you go vegan, there's not going to be anything good to eat around the house anymore. This is incredibly selfish of you." (You can tell him to go screw himself. In the most loving way, of course.) Or your mother might ask, "Are you insinuating that your father and I were bad parents by feeding you meat? How dare you!"

If you get responses like this, just reassure your family that you're not trying to make them miserable and you're not judging them. Tell them you still love them as much as when you were eating hamburgers together, but you've just decided to make a new choice based on new information. If you deliver that message in a compassionate and loving tone, they will respect it, even if they still don't "get it."

No matter what sort of comments you get, going vegan doesn't need to become an issue in your relationships. When my ex-wife Kimora Lee and I were first married, she wasn't interested in giving up animal products. And that was fine. I had my refrigerator with all my vegan food in it, and she had hers with her meat and dairy. There wasn't any tension or resentment. She ate what she wanted to eat, and I did the same. Separate refrigerators might not be an option for everyone, but no matter what your situation is, you can work out a compromise.

Take my brother Rev Run. I've tried to get him to give up animal products for years but to no avail. He even just started hosting a cooking show where he makes steaks and pork chops. I wish he would cook something else, but that doesn't mean we love each other any less. He still comes over to my house to eat and I go over to his. We might tease each other a bit, but we're still brothers. I am very happy to say that Rev's daughter Angela has become a vegan. That doesn't mean she and her father have issues. They're actually incredibly close, and he supports her choice completely. Even if he hasn't made it himself—yet (I'm not giving up hope).

I'm blessed to be part of an especially supportive family, so we've been able get past whatever little bumps we've encountered. Yours might be trickier. The pushback you get might knock you off stride a bit. If you feel like you're not getting the support you need from those closest to you, what I would strongly suggest is seeking out a community of vegans or vegetarians where you live and soaking up some of their energy.

In Los Angeles and New York City, that's going to be easy. Those cities have vibrant communities and all sorts of great options in groceries, restaurants, and services to choose from. A friend of mine who moved from Turkey to L.A. a couple of years ago said that she'd never heard about a vegan diet before coming to L.A. Now she finds herself around so many people who don't eat animal products that she says she feels "a little weird *not* being a vegan."

Outside of Los Angeles and New York, attitudes can still be less accepting. I have a friend who follows a pescatarian diet (someone who doesn't eat meat but does consume dairy and fish). She lives in L.A. too and says no one there bats an eye if she tells them about her diet. If anything, people might ask her, "Why don't you go all the way vegan?"

But when she goes home to Chicago and mentions she doesn't eat meat, people look at her like she's crazy. Friends have asked her—in all seriousness—if she's joined a cult. Or if she's sick. This is Chicago we're talking about. The third-largest city in America.

I don't want to create the impression that if you're not in L.A. or NYC it's going to be impossible to go vegan. Cities like San Francisco, Philadelphia, New Orleans, Boston, San Diego, and Miami all have thriving vegan scenes. As do college towns like Austin, Texas; Madison,

Wisconsin; Amherst, Massachusetts; and Ann Arbor, Michigan. Young people, thankfully, are much more open-minded about and conscious of the food they put in their bodies than their parents were.

But if you don't live in one of these places, then yes, you might have to work a little bit harder to make connections. You're going to have to seek people out—either online or in person. Join a Facebook group of vegans and get alerts every time a new green grocery store opens up in your area. Share posts about an Indian place you've discovered that has terrific curry, or the Chinese spot that has the best eggplant dishes. Find out where other vegans are eating. Even try to organize a meet-up or group dinner with other vegans in your area.

Perhaps most important, remember that just because you join a vegan community, it doesn't mean you have to reject any other ones. I love to hang out at vegan restaurants, but that doesn't mean I'm not going to come to your birthday party if you have it at a restaurant that serves meat. My friend recently had a party at a steakhouse in L.A. and of course I showed up. I just told the waitress to bring me the biggest salad they had with a side of sautéed spinach. Everyone was eating steaks around me, but I didn't feel like I was missing out. Nor did I give them a hard time for eating meat. We were there to enjoy each other's company and that's what we did. No matter what the situation, I try to live my truth and hope it inspires the people around me to make a similar choice.

One of the keys to both my success and my happiness is feeling like I'm connected with as many different kinds of people as possible. The other day I was back in NYC and started my day with a hot yoga class, where probably over half the people were vegans.

After my class, I paid a visit to my old stomping grounds in Hollis. I was on the corner for only few minutes before I was chopping it up with a lot of guys I grew up with. We reminisced about little schemes we used to run, girls we used to mess with, and rival crews we used to fight. It felt great to be around my old friends again.

On the surface those two scenes might seem like they were worlds apart. A hot yoga class in Manhattan and a hot corner in Hollis. But I felt completely comfortable in both spaces. I loved the vibes I got at yoga that morning, just as I loved soaking up the energy of my old hood.

I love feeling connected with people from different walks of life, even if to the outside world there doesn't seem to be any connection between them. That's why I'm going to keep hanging with vegans, just like I'm going to keep hanging with my Hollis crew. Just like I'm going to keep hanging with my rabbi friends and my Nation of Islam friends too. My friends might have different opinions or practices or diets, but that doesn't mean you can't be part of all of their worlds. If I were to start hanging with only vegans or Jews or old-school hustlers, life would get boring fast. But by moving between different worlds, I'm always exposed to new ideas and perspectives. It helps keep me young and inspired. And if I can, in turn, expose some people to the benefits of giving up animal products, then I can help them feel better too.

GIVING UP MEAT IS FOR ANIMAL LOVERS

"The greatness of a nation and its moral progress can be judged by the way its animals are treated." —GANDHI

It's funny, I was recently telling a friend about this book, and she was inspired when I told her about how giving up meat would help improve her health. She was incredulous when I told her how much the meat and dairy industries hurt the environment. Yet when I started talking to her about the horrible suffering inflicted on factory-farmed animals, suddenly she changed her tune. "Russell, I'm not interested in all that PETA stuff," she said, waving her hand. "I'm not one of your little animal-loving friends."

This is a pretty common reaction. If you're not a "weirdo" or a "freak" for giving up animal products, then you must be an "animal lover" who has lost all sense of perspective. Not that there's anything wrong with that, but I had to laugh because I am not what you might consider a stereotypical "animal lover."

Don't get it twisted—I'm extremely proud and grateful that in 2011 PETA named me their Man of the Year. Out of all the awards that have been given to me over the years, it's among the ones I treasure most.

Still, you're not going to see me out on the street throwing paint on rich ladies' mink coats. My style is to try to educate people about the choices they're making. I still attend fashion shows that feature fur, something many in the vegan community won't do. Though I do always make a point to try to speak to the designer afterward and let him or her know that there's no reason to still be using real fur. I made some headlines following a Michael Kors show when I tweeted, "Michael Kors so talented. Beautiful clothes. Too much fur. Kinda hurts to sit thru." I'm sure he didn't appreciate it, but I hope it inspired him to check out some of the Japanese faux fur—which is really very beautiful and feels great—that's now available to designers.

Simone, on the other hand, would never sit through a fashion show that featured fur. She's unbelievably invested in working with organizations like PETA, Mercy for Animals, Farm Sanctuary, and Social Compassion in Legislation to stop the abuse of farm animals. Since she started working for me in the early days of Def Jam Records, Simone has been giving lectures, raising funds, and personally saving dozens of animals. I stopped counting all the birds with broken wings she's brought home over the years.

When you come to my house, however, you won't see any birds on the mend. Or rescue dogs or cats. But there's still room for both of us in the community. Simone is currently taking care of a blind rescue dog named Hubbell Yoda, which she brings to the office with her every day. (It's one of the funniest-looking creatures you've ever seen—lots of fluffy hair and nothing but fur where its eyes should be.) Even though that dog has been sitting in my office every day for the past few years, I never even tried to pet it. I'm just not that into dogs. Or cats or birds, for that matter.

> "I think Russell helps debunk the myth of what it means to be an 'animal activist.' It's true, I bring Hubbell Yoda to the office with us every day and he goes on trips with us too. Russell is around Yoda 24/7. You know how many times Russell has reached down and petted him (unless it's for a photo shoot)? Zero! Never! And that's fine. Because being a vegan isn't about being an animal lover. It's about being compassionate. And believing in social justice."
>
> —Simone Reyes

But just because I don't happen to want to be an animal *lover* doesn't meant that I want to be an animal *killer*. Just because I don't want to pet blind rescue dogs or have a cat for a companion doesn't mean I'm OK being part of a system that causes suffering for billions of other living creatures.

As I'll explain later, one of my primary goals in life is to be compassionate. And it's impossible to be a compassionate person if you eat animal products.

So if you're like my friend and want me to miss you with "all the PETA stuff," know that attitude is a cop-out. If you put this meat and dairy in your body every day, then you need to confront the reality that you are contributing to a system of suffering. What you do after you confront those realities is up to you.

I'M NO GOOD AT GOING ON DIETS

> *"Our bodies are designed to remain in balance, and when they go out of balance, a natural mechanism has been interfered with."* —DEEPAK CHOPRA

Not good at going on diets?

Not a problem because this isn't a diet book.

There is a good chance you will lose weight when you embrace a plant-based diet—as I said, I lost about twenty pounds. J. Lo said she lost twelve. Beyoncé and my niece Angela both definitely slimmed down after giving up animal products. The list could go on and on. Still, losing weight is not even remotely the goal of this book.

My goal in these pages is to help you change your *lifestyle*. I want to help you build a more graceful, healthier, happier, and compassionate relationship with the world. Not just help you fit into a new dress. Or fit into "skinny jeans." If those are the changes you're looking for, then you're probably going to want to pick up another book.

I'm aware losing weight is a priority for a lot of folks—studies have shown almost half the country is on one sort of diet or another. Yet despite all that calorie counting, weight watching, and carb cutting, almost 80 percent of people who lose weight on diets end up gaining it back. In a lot of ways, going on a diet is like going on a vacation. Yes, you might go somewhere that looks and feels better, but you usually end up right back where you started.

That sort of up-and-down relationship with what you eat is known as "yo-yo dieting," and it can be incredibly discouraging. You spend a couple of weeks, or maybe months, enjoying the "new you" and then just as quickly you find yourself back at your old weight. Or even heavier. After that happens a few times, it can become very tempting to tell yourself, "I'm never going to be able to lose weight" and then resign yourself to a life of unhealthy eating.

When you make a lifestyle change, you're going to cut the cord to that yo-yo. When you change your lifestyle, whether you gain a few pounds here or lose a few pounds there becomes immaterial. No matter what the scale says, you know you are healthier. You know whether your pants feel snug or not but you'll also know that you are doing your part to help the environment. You might be a few pounds over your high school weight, but you feel great because your karma is no longer connected to the abuse of the animals.

MEDITATION AND YOGA

> "Through the practices of yoga, we discover that concern for
> the happiness and well-being of others, including animals,
> must be an essential part of our own quest for happiness and
> well-being. The fork can be a powerful weapon of mass de-
> struction or a tool to create peace on Earth."
>
> —SHARON GANNON

You probably weren't expecting a section on yoga and meditation in a vegan book, but there's simply no way I could encourage you to give up animal products without telling you about what I consider to be the two best tools for the job.

I've met people who said they tried a vegan diet, but claimed it didn't stick. They were committed for a moment, but then drifted back to their old (bad) habits. They might blame their relapse on a number of factors—time, money, taste, acceptance—but I don't buy those excuses. To me, it all comes down to mindfulness. When you can approach your *entire* life—not just your diet—mindfully, you're going to be able to make the right decisions and stick to them. When you're distracted, it'll always be an uphill battle.

We talk about states of consciousness like enlightenment, Nirvana, and Christ consciousness as if they were almost unattainable goals, but the truth is you already possess them in your heart. You just have to remember to access them. Yoga, meditation, and a plant-based diet will help you do that.

Stepping out of a yoga class after spending an hour sweating and twisting, you can suddenly have a sense of being alive like you've never experienced before: When you say, "Oh my god, what an amazing experience" and feel like you're awake for the first time. For example, you can spend twenty minutes meditating and actually feel your mind reboot. Or eat one healthy meal and realize that you prefer feeling lifted up instead of slowed down.

To be clear, yoga, meditation, and a plant-based diet are all helpful on their own. But when you can combine all three practices into your lifestyle, it's going to speed up your evolution significantly.

No matter how old you are, or what you do, your goal should be to move through life in the most graceful and least harmful way possible. That's it. Yoga promotes this. Too many of the other physical practices that are popular in America don't.

For instance, everyone seems to think that the best way to get in shape is by going to the gym and lifting weights. But do you know what you do when you lift weights? You rip your muscle fibers apart. That might make you look ripped in the short term, but in the long term it's not healthy for your body. Every physical activity you do should be about lengthening your muscles and promoting circulation, not making your muscles tighter and thicker.

It's the same with running. Everyone thinks they have to jog a couple miles every day to stay in shape or lose weight, but forcing your knees, ankles, and feet to absorb all that repetitive pounding isn't a helpful solution. Running puts your body through a lot of abuse without offering any sort of long-term gain.

Yoga, on the other hand, isn't about ripping, pounding, or cracking. It's not about beating your body up. Instead, yoga heals the body through promoting circulation. When you sit on the yoga mat and focus on twisting and lengthening your muscles, you will feel the blood and energy begin to circulate around your body. That movement is what is going to keep you healthy over the long run.

For thousands of years, the yogis have taught that no sickness can live in a body that has constant circulation. That might seem like a lofty claim, but the more you practice yoga, the more you'll realize how true it is. The key to a happy and graceful life is circulation. It's about listening to your body and learning how to breathe energy into the parts that need it. It's about learning how to lengthen your body instead of ripping it apart or pounding it into the ground.

All that grunting, panting, and pushing isn't really doing you any good. That's not how you want to move through life. That's why I put the picture of me in a yogi pose on the cover of this book. Do I look beat up or run down? Of course not. I'm giggling in that picture because getting into that pose, no matter how difficult it might look, was fun. I'm happy in that picture because I've realized how cool it is to move through life with the least amount of harm possible.

As you move through life, please make sure every practice and habit that's part of your lifestyle promotes lengthening and circulation, not stiffness and blockage.

Meat in your digestive track blocks circulation. A vegan diet promotes circulation. Lifting weights shortens and stiffens your muscles. Yoga lengthens your muscles. Even social media, as much as we love it, shortens our interactions with the world. Meditation lengthens the moments and promotes clarity.

This lifestyle I'm promoting—one centered around a plant-based diet, meditation, and yoga—is designed to lengthen your life. To lengthen animals' lives. To lengthen Mother Earth's life.

It might seem to be very different from your current lifestyle, but I promise once you get a taste of it, you're not going to want to do anything to foul it up. If you used to drink a lot, you're not going to want to wake up with a hangover anymore. If you used to do drugs, you're not going to want to have a cloudy brain anymore. And if you used to eat animal products, you're not going to want to keep compromising your circulation (to say nothing of your karma) anymore either.

I still remember the exact moment I realized that. I was taking a yoga class led by Dechen Thurman, the brother of the actress Uma Thurman and son of the Buddhist scholar Robert Thurman. It was a really intense class that had me doing all these twists and difficult poses. With each one, I could almost feel the toxins and bad energy being wrung out of my body. My shirt was absolutely soaked with sweat. Before sending us back out into the world, Dechen ended the class with this instruction: "Now go out there and put something into your body that fuels your practice and makes it better. Not slows it down."

When he said this, it was as if someone had rung a bell in my head. I was feeling so alive and free in the moment that all I could imagine myself ever eating again was vegetable juice and maybe a piece of kale.

Eating anything else, especially animal products, seemed like it would be mainlining poison right into my system. The idea of ingesting meat into my body, where it would sit and rot in my veins for months, ran counter to everything I had just experienced in that class.

Practicing yoga is going to help you see the benefits of promoting circulation and help steer you away from anything that might compromise that. Trust me, your body is not happy when it has animal products rotting away inside of it, and it tries to let you know. It tries to let you know by making you sluggish after you eat a steak. It tries to let you know by making you feel cramped and bloated when you drink cow's milk. Just like it tries to let you know with a heart attack.

Too many of us, unfortunately, don't heed those warnings until it's almost too late. When you practice yoga, however, you're going to hear what your body is telling you loud and clear from almost the first day you start your practice. When you sit on that mat for the first time and begin to reconnect with your body, you're going to feel just how stiff and rigid you've become. Over time, as you build your practice and that stiffness gives way to fluidity and gracefulness, you're not going to want to do anything or ingest anything that's going to take you back to that rigid place. This is why I always say that yoga and veganism go hand in hand.

I know when many of you think of yoga, you probably picture people doing poses or stretches on mats in a class. But those poses, or *asanas* as they're known in Sanskrit, are actually only one branch of a much larger tree that makes up yoga. I'm going to list all those separate branches in a sidebar, but I want to take a moment to explain why it was so important to me to include the laws of yoga in a book about veganism.

Many of us are stuck in cycles of negative behavior. Eating animals is just one of them. You could be stuck in a cycle of dysfunctional relationships, a cycle of drug abuse, a cycle of aimlessness, or a cycle of insecurity. No matter what cycle you're stuck in, these laws are designed to help you stop on a dime and move in a different direction.

They were compiled thousands of years ago in a book called the *Yoga Sūtras of Patañjali*, but they're as effective today as they were when they were first written down. I've read the translation by Swami Satchidananda many times, and I'm always struck by how effective a tool these sutras are. I think their greatest gift is teaching us how to live in the present instead of worrying about the past. Just because the world roughed you up a bit in the past doesn't mean you have to be fearful of the future. The sutras teach us how to step out of that fearful mind state and jump into the present.

And for anyone who might feel funny about exploring laws that are rooted in yoga, please understand that yoga isn't a religion. It's a scientific approach to obtaining happiness and enlightenment. It can be practiced by Christians, Jews, Muslims, or people of any religion. And I think when you explore the laws, you'll find they echo the teachings of the Judeo-Christian tradition very closely.

THE EIGHT STEPS OF CLASSICAL YOGA

1. Yama: Universal morality, represented by five separate branches of the yogic tree:

- Ahimsa: compassion for all living things
- Satya: non-lying and respect for the truth
- Asteya: non-stealing and detachment from belief that possessions can create happiness
- Brahmacharya: abstention from "harmful" sex and emotional manipulation
- Aparigraha: non-greed and letting go of attachments

2. Niyama: Personal observances and social laws. These are also broken down into five parts:

- Sauca: purity
- Santosa: contentment
- Tapas: energy to burn through life's distractions
- Svadhyaya: self-reflection
- Isvarapranidhana: surrendering to the spiritual self

3. Asana (or Seat): Body poses and the physical practice of yoga

4. Pranayama: Breathing exercises and the control of life force

5. Pratyahara: Control of the senses

6. Dharana: Concentration on one's purpose in life

7. Dhyana: Meditation and devotion on the divine

8. Samadhi: Union with the divine

The other practice I've found that goes hand in hand with being a vegan is meditation. Like yoga, meditation helps pull you out of your distracted state and allows you to reconnect with your body and your mind. It's said, and I believe, that there's a piece of God inside all of us. When we meditate, we get to touch that piece.

Doing so allows us to reconnect with the needs of both our body and our spirit. When you sit in silence in meditation, it allows you to shut out all the noise of the world and hear God's instructions on what is healthy and unhealthy.

A distracted mind is much more likely to be tripped up by all the bullshit out there in the world. It's not so much that we choose to do dumb or hurtful things. It's more that we ignore that voice of God telling us not to do them.

When you meditate, however, it becomes impossible to ignore that voice. When you sit in silence every day, instead of getting your instructions from the world, you get them from the spirit. As a person who is nonreligious but deeply spiritual, I believe that should be our goal in life. To move according to the spirit, instead of the world.

When you move according to the spirit, it's almost impossible to make harmful, selfish choices. There's no way someone who meditates every day could ever decide to say, "I support slavery," or "I support throwing people in ovens."

Just as I believe there's no way someone who meditates every day could ever support eating animal products. If you sat and meditated for twenty minutes about the suffering of the animals, you'd probably start to cry. That you'd stand up, go back out into the world, and decide to eat a steak would be virtually impossible.

In his book *How to Eat*, the Buddhist monk Thích Nhất Hạnh writes that when it comes to our food choices, we must remember that "nothing comes from nothing." In other words, we can't forget that a drumstick was once the leg of a live chicken. That a sirloin steak was once the back of a live steer. When you're *distracted*, your mind won't always make the connection between the living, breathing cow that was brutally slaughtered and that piece of pink meat wrapped in plastic you just bought at the grocery store. But when you use meditation to slow down your mind, that connection is going to be very clear.

Paul McCartney says making that sort of connection is what made him stop eating animal products. "Many years ago, I was fishing, and as I was reeling in the poor fish, I realized, 'I am killing him—all for the passing pleasure it brings me.'" I don't think it's a coincidence that McCartney has also been a meditator for many years.

In addition to helping you make better choices, yoga and meditation also both build discipline. Yoga and meditation have transformed my life, but I had to develop a lot of self-control to practice them every day. For fifteen years, I've meditated every morning as soon as I wake up, but there are still plenty of times where I'd much rather hit the snooze button and go back to bed for another twenty minutes. Just as there are plenty of afternoons where I'm working on a new TV or film project and I don't feel like dropping everything so that I can rush off to my 6:30 hot yoga class. Still, I honor my commitment every time because I know that thirty seconds into that meditation I'll feel so peaceful. Or that after spending an hour sweating like a slave in hot yoga, I'm going to stand up and feel like I'm in heaven.

As I said, I'm not a religious person, but I do follow those practices religiously. I'd rather be late to a breakfast meeting than skip my morning meditation. My assistants are constantly tinkering with my schedule, but they know that my yoga is nonnegotiable. There's no deal, no meeting, no conference call that's more important to me than taking the time to go to class and get my body and mind right. I know that ultimately I can accomplish a lot more with the grace and peace that come from yoga and meditation than with the frustration and anxiety that result from rushing unconsciously through your day.

No matter how you arrive at the decision to cut animal products out of your diet—concerns about your health, fears for the environment, or outrage over the treatment of the animals—a lifestyle switch of that magnitude might feel intimidating at first. Meditation and yoga will help you find the courage and discipline to take the first steps. They say that learning the guitar is easier if you know the piano first. I believe it's the same with yoga and meditation and giving up animal products. If you incorporate them into your lifestyle first, removing animal products will be a much smoother transition.

If you don't already practice yoga, please check out a class. Don't be intimidated if you don't feel like you can do the physical poses—or asanas—as well as everyone else at first. Unlike many of the physical activities we practice in America, yoga is not competitive. The teacher isn't going to yell at you if you can't keep up. In fact, one of the first things you'll often hear when you walk into class is, "Please leave your ego and your shoes at the door." Yoga isn't about doing better than the person on the mat next to you. It's about reconnecting with *your* body and *your* spirit. You could do that through performing every pose the teacher asks of you or you could do it by sitting in the same position for the entire class.

There's literally no reason—physically, spiritually, or financially—not to check out a yoga class. They're fairly cheap (most classes range from $10 to $20) and yoga studios can be found in most places around the country today. If for some reason you can't find a class where you live, there are many excellent yoga apps and DVDs that allow you to practice at home. In terms of what type of class to attend, these days I'm doing a lot of hot yoga, where they heat the room up to over a hundred degrees. I love how the heat gets my circulation flowing and makes it even easier to lengthen my limbs, but it might not be the style everyone is comfortable starting with. If you're a beginner, you might want to check out a Hatha or Vinyasa class, which represent the most basic yoga styles. Then as you become more comfortable, you can play around with some other styles until you find the ones that fit best for you.

As for meditation, I recommend a mantra-based practice. It's the style I detailed in my book *Success Through Stillness* and the one I've found is most effective for beginners. If you didn't read that book or just feel you need a refresher, I include a step-by-step guide to meditation at the end of this book.

Ultimately, a lot of practices can help you find the sense of stillness and clarity that meditation promotes. Mantra-based meditation is one but so is candle gazing (which is just what it sounds like). You might be able to get that clarity from a practice like qigong, or even gardening.

No matter how you arrive there, you want a lifestyle that's clear, not cloudy. That's sensitive instead of disconnected. Where making helpful, compassionate choices comes naturally and hurtful actions feel wrong immediately.

It's a lifestyle you might arrive at from "just" being a yogi, "just" being a meditator, or "just" being a vegan. But if you can incorporate all three of these practices into your daily routine, there's simply no way that in a short time you won't find yourself living the happiest and healthiest lifestyle possible.

GIVING UP MEAT WILL MAKE ME WEAK

> *"Being vegan improved my performance off and on the field. . . . You're able to take more energy from plant-based sources than animal-based sources. The list goes on, and it translates to the field and how I recover."*
>
> —MONTELL OWENS, NFL RUNNING BACK

Another common excuse I hear people fall back on is that they think giving up meat will make them weak. I've heard plenty of women make comments like, "If I give up meat I'll look too stringy," or "Those girls who don't eat meat don't look right. They look gray." I have to chuckle whenever I hear talk like that. A woman can see another woman with a double chin, stomach fat, back boobs, and greasy skin yet never make a comment about her diet. But if she sees a female vegan who has a bit of pallor or, God forbid, is a little skinny, then that becomes a serious judgment against the whole vegan lifestyle.

I don't know where those gray or washed-out comments come from, because the vast majority of vegan women I know of look absolutely incredible. In addition to carrying less weight, most of the vegan women I've met have smoother and brighter skin than those who eat animal products. (The only way going vegan might negatively affect your skin is if you start eating or juicing a ton of carrots. In that case, your skin can take on a slightly orange tint, and it means it's time to cut back.)

Have you seen Jennifer Lopez lately? I did, not too long ago, in person, and she was absolutely glowing. She practically lit up the entire room with her energy.

> "I enjoy eating that way. I never did. And I didn't know how good you can feel when you put healthy stuff in your body."
> —Jennifer Lopez on adopting a plant-based diet

J. Lo says that thanks to her plant-based diet she was able to shed her post-baby weight in just a matter of weeks. "I'll be honest, since I had the babies about six years ago, I had that really stubborn eight to ten pounds on me," she told *Extra*. "People are used to seeing me be kind of thickish, but when I started eating [vegan], right away I dropped like eight to ten pounds." J. Lo also says she loved how her energy and focus improved. "It was a real change, but more than that I felt better and people were like, 'Your energy's better' . . . everything's better."

It's the same with Beyoncé. Did you see any articles about Bey not looking right or losing any of her trademark fierceness when she went on her vegan challenge? Of course not. When Beyoncé gave up animal products, she kept looking as powerful and fabulous as ever. She even told the *New York Times* that she had "a noticeable glow to my skin" after taking her vegan challenge.

"The benefits of a plant-based diet need to be known. We should spend more time loving ourselves, which means taking better care of ourselves with good nutrition and making healthier food choices."

—Beyoncé

Venus Williams is another great example. Does Venus look unhealthy to you? Is her body "too stringy"? I didn't think so. Well, Venus gave up animal products back in 2011. She made the change after being diagnosed with Sjögren's syndrome, an autoimmune disease that had been leaving her fatigued, short of breath, and experiencing a lot of muscle pain. Venus says that since giving up animal products and dairy her symptoms have improved and that changing her diet has made a "big difference" in improving her tennis game. The year after giving up animal products, Venus and her sister Serena won the doubles championships at both the Olympics and Wimbledon. I guess giving up animal products didn't make her too weak, huh?

Men need to understand that there's no connection between animal products and physical vitality either. Too many men have been tricked into believing that without a constant supply of animal products in their diet, they'd somehow be sapped of their Herculean strength and would shrivel up into little raisins.

I'm not even going to address whether a lot of those guys are even as strong as they'd like to believe they are, but just as Venus has continued to excel at her sport while eating a plant-based diet, it needs to be said that there are plenty of male professional athletes who have made the same choice. And experienced the same results.

Former NFL star Tony Gonzalez decided to eat a plant-based diet after reading a book called *The China Study*, which I'll discuss more in the next chapter. After almost completely eliminating animal products from his diet in 2008, he went on to catch ten touchdown passes, one of the best totals for his career. "I have more energy, better focus, and more endurance. I don't get tired," he told *Men's Journal* at the time. "I hardly ever come out of the game. And I'm strong as ever."

Gonzalez also found that eliminating animal products cut down on inflammation (something a lot of meat eaters experience) and helped him better handle the injuries that are part of life in the NFL. "Eating a more plant-based diet has allowed me to bounce back quicker, it's helped me to stay around the NFL and still play at the high-level I play at—at a physically demanding position. I attribute everything to my diet," he told MindBodyGreen. (In an ironic twist, in 2009 Gonzalez also made headlines after he performed the Heimlich maneuver on a diner choking to death in a restaurant. What was the guy choking on? You guessed it, a piece of meat.)

Gonzalez isn't the only NFL player to experience success on and off the field after giving up animal products. The running back Ricky Williams played five successful seasons in the NFL after becoming a vegetarian. "It changed my game, and it changed my body," he told *Men's Journal*. "I had tons of energy."

Georges Laraque went vegan while starring in the National Hockey League, where he was known for his powerful style of play. "I have never felt better or so healthy in my life," says Laraque, whose parents immigrated to Canada from Haiti. "Rest assured that there are tons of proteins in vegetarian products that are much better for your health because vegetarian products aren't filled with the cholesterol that animal protein is filled with."

OK, so far we've got a tennis champion, two NFL stars, and a NHL tough guy all saying that a vegan diet, far from hurting them, has actually improved their strength, endurance, and ability to compete. Still not convinced? Well, check out what mixed martial arts champion Mac Danzig has to say about going vegan. Because they don't come much tougher than MMA fighters.

"When I decided to go vegan, I was able to make [weight] much easier, and I haven't lost an ounce of muscle," Danzig says in the excellent documentary *Forks Over Knives*. "I'm leaner than I used to be, and I have much more energy than I used to."

In an interview with the Ultimate Fighting Championship (UFC), Danzig explains that while he loves the extra energy being a vegan brings him in the ring, his decision to give up animal products wasn't just about improved performance:

At the very beginning for me it was moral and ethical. In this day and age, buying animal and dairy products causes way more suffering and harm than it does good. Don't get me wrong, yes, I love animals . . . but if we were in a different day and age, like 100 or 200 years ago, then, sure, I would do whatever I had to do to live. If I had to be a hunter-gatherer then I would. I might feel bad about it, but I would respect the animals that I killed and I would eat meat. But things are different. We don't live in that day and age anymore. Today you have processed meats and a lot of animals suffering unnecessarily for it.

Now, some people just blow that off and don't have a conscience about it or they just don't care. They wouldn't eat their dog but they feel that way about other animals. But for me, I just decided to stop eating meat. I didn't want to contribute to all of that. I'm not trying to change the world or wear that on my sleeve or make a political statement, because that just turns people away. I only have control over one person and that's myself. And I feel good about it.

Danzing's story is a powerful reminder that physical strength and compassion aren't mutually exclusive. That it is possible to excel in a sport as physically demanding as mixed martial arts without sacrificing either your strength or your integrity. Today, people like Danzing might still be considered outliers. But I'm confident that in the not-too-distant future more and more athletes will follow his lead. No wonder the UFC, the epicenter of America's tough-guy culture, calls Danzing, "a pioneer who was ahead of the times."

STRONGER AT WHATEVER YOU DO

Physical strength is great, but I want to talk about other ways your strength will improve when you give up animal products.

There's no doubt that giving up animal products has made me much stronger and more effective as an entrepreneur. A lot of success in business depends on bringing a consistent level of focus and determination day in and day out. As Woody Allen once said, "Eighty percent of success is just showing up."

I might not always make the right call on a new start-up or come up with an idea that's going to turn a company around overnight, but if there's one thing you can say about me as a businessman, it's that I show up every day. No matter where I am or what's happening in my life, I follow the same script. Again, I might not be religious, but I practice my lifestyle religiously. Every day, I'm up at 5:30 to meditate. After a shower and a green juice, I head over to my ex-wife's and meditate again with my kids before I take them to school. I'm at the office by nine, and work straight through to my 6:30 yoga. After that, I go home and then get back to work again until 10:00 or so at night. It's a pretty intense schedule, yet I rarely feel like I'm dragging. I never have a moment in the morning when I say, "Man, I don't feel like going to work today." Just as I never come home thinking, "I'm tired of this shit." Instead, I wake up every day looking forward to whatever is going to come across my desk. How many people in their late fifties can say that? Let alone in their thirties or forties? I'm convinced that there's no way I could keep up that pace every day if I were still eating animal products. Before I made the switch I can remember going out to lunch and having a burger or a big plate of ribs and feeling like I was in a fog when I got back to the office. Sometimes I'd be so tired that I'd have to head to the Russian baths for a steam so I could rest and "recover" from what I just ate. By the time I'd get out of there, half my afternoon would be gone. That's not the recipe for a successful day.

Now I finish my lunch and actually feel *more* energized. It's like a power boost to propel me through the second half of my day. Can you say that about your lunch? Do you come back to your office feeling refreshed and ready to tackle everything that's still on your to-do list? Or do you come back feeling like you need a nap? If your answer is "nap," take a look at what you're putting in your body. If you're eating a hamburger or a chicken Parm sub during lunch, that stuff is going to slow you down. You'll be at your desk dragging, while the person next to you, who had a salad and piece of fruit, is already going to be off and running. If that's the case every day, you tell me who is more likely to get promoted first. Who is more likely to land the bigger account? Who is more likely to catch their boss's eye? It's going to be the person with the most energy who is maximizing their time to the fullest.

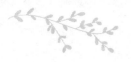

HEALTH THROUGH
A PLANT-BASED DIET

> *"Some people think the plant-based, whole-foods diet is extreme. Half a million people a year will have their chests opened up and a vein taken from their leg and sewn onto their coronary artery. Some people would call that extreme."* —DR. CALDWELL ESSELSTYN

Now that I've cleared up some of the misconceptions on why you *can't* go vegan, I want to address the main reasons you *should*.

Let's start with your health, because I believe that getting your own body together should always be your first priority. I talk a lot about the importance of being a great servant, but it's almost impossible to help anyone else if your own well-being isn't firmly established. You know when they announce the safety instructions on an airplane, they always tell you to put on your own oxygen mask before you try to help someone else with theirs? I view a person's relationship with the world the same way. I can't ask you to protect the environment, or help save the animals if you don't have your own body together first.

The importance of taking care of yourself first is a concept I learned through yoga, where it's taught that you must get your root chakra (or *Muladhara*) together first before you can take care of the remaining ones. If you're not familiar with them, chakras are seven energy sources that run from the base of your spine to the top of your head (see the chart on the next page). When they're aligned properly, your relationship with the world is going to be in a healthy balance. You're going to be happier and healthier and have more energy. When those chakras aren't flowing correctly, you're going to be jammed up and out of whack. You'll be more likely to feel depressed and be susceptible to illnesses.

In addition to practices like yoga and meditation, giving up animal products is a very effective way to keep that root chakra flowing freely.

You might not even be aware of it, but the animal products you ingest are slowing you down. They're going to decrease your metabolism and make you gain weight. They're sitting in your digestive track, rotting away and sapping you of critical energy. In the short term, they're going to make you feel sluggish. In the long term, they're going to potentially make you very, very sick.

But only if you let them.

For too long, there was a popular perception that we didn't have much say about our long-term health. That conditions like heart disease, cancer, and Alzheimer's were largely due to genetics. We believed that we got prostate cancer because our father had it or we developed high blood pressure because it ran in the family. As crazy as it might sound, there was something almost reassuring in believing that.

Why worry about eating steak every night if you're probably going to have high blood pressure anyway? Why bother cutting out dairy if breast cancer is just "something the women in our family get"?

THE SEVEN CHAKRAS

1. **Root chakra, or Muladhara:** Our foundation of being grounded and secure

Location: Base of spine

2. **Sacral chakra, or Svadhisthana:** Ability to accept new things and experiences, especially creatively

Location: Lower abdomen

3. **Solar plexus chakra, or Manipura:** Feeling confident and personally in control

Location: Upper abdomen

4. **Heart chakra, or Anahata:** Our ability to love and be connected; our bridge between the physical and spiritual selves

Location: Center of chest above the heart

5. **Throat chakra, or Vishuddha:** Ability to communicate and share

Location: Throat

6. **Third-eye chakra, or Ajna:** Ability to focus on big picture and intuition

Location: Forehead between the eyes

7. **Crown chakra, or Sahaswara:** The highest, the ability to be fully connected

Location: Top of the head

Today we know we have a stronger say in our health. Yes, there are some conditions you might develop from genetics, bad luck, or even both. Most of the deadly killers lurking out there, however, are conditions that you can not only avoid but also reverse—through your diet. If fifty years ago we thought that diseases like cancer were caused 70 percent by genetics and 30 percent by environment, today we know the opposite is true.

> "Each generation of medical students learns about a different set of pills and procedures, but receives almost no training in disease prevention. And in practice, doctors are not rewarded for educating patients about the merits of truly healthy lifestyles."
> —Dr. Caldwell Esselstyn

In the plainest terms, now we know that you can kill yourself by eating the wrong stuff and heal yourself by eating the right stuff. And the wrong stuff is animal products, while the right stuff is vegetables and other plant-based foods. No doctor or nutritionist, if they're being honest, can be unclear about that.

Unfortunately, this truth isn't reflected in how we practice medicine in this country. Instead of helping people make the healthiest choices with their food a priority, we're focused on what happens *after* you get sick. We've created a system in this country where our doctors are more focused on giving you a pill or making you undergo a procedure than actually addressing the root of what's making you sick.

Nine times out of ten, if you see a doctor about high blood pressure or high cholesterol levels, he or she is going to prescribe you a pill. Sure, your doctor'll probably encourage you to cut down on sodium, but the prescription pad is probably already out while she's saying it. It's not because your doctor is being lazy; prescribing pills for conditions is what doctors have been taught to do.

We've accepted a system where spending your life dependent on pills, or even *cutting open your chest*, seems like a more practical choice than *cutting out animal products* from your diet. Think about that.

As a country, we keep getting richer and more technologically advanced. So it would stand to reason that we should be getting healthier too, right? Sadly just the opposite is true.

More than one-third of Americans are overweight. That number is projected to increase by more than 40 percent by 2030. Deadly diseases like cancer, heart disease, and diabetes are all on the rise. In fact, Americans have twice the diabetes rate and three times the cancer rate than the rest of the world.

How could such an affluent, progressive country like ours keep getting fatter and fatter? And sicker and sicker? Because of what we eat. Instead of building our diets on healthy, nutritious, plant-based foods that prevent disease, we've built them on animal products, which actually encourage sickness and disease.

What I hope you'll get from this chapter is that you don't have to go down the same path as everyone else. Your future doesn't rest in the hands of your genes. Or luck. Instead, I want you to embrace the concept that *your* choices are going to be the greatest factor in determining how well and how long you're going to live.

HEART DISEASE

> *"Last year over a million people left the same suicide note . . . Shopping List: butter, eggs, milk, beef, and bacon."*
> —PHYSICIANS COMMITTEE FOR RESPONSIBLE MEDICINE

I first started working on this book while the Ebola hysteria was reaching a crescendo. Every time I turned on my TV or computer, I'd be greeted by updates about the latest outbreak. Politicians were suggesting shutting the airports, people stopped going to work, parents kept their kids out of school, and everyone seemed to take all of these crazy precautions.

Then in a few weeks, it was all over. One person had died, several more had been hospitalized, but that was it. Of course in countries like Liberia, Sierra Leone, and Senegal the situation continues to be very grave, but in America the amount of media attention and public outcry didn't match the actual impact of Ebola on the population.

Compare the breathless Ebola coverage to how much attention we pay to heart disease, which actually *is* the number one killer in this country. According to the Centers for Disease Control and Prevention (CDC), heart disease is responsible for six hundred thousand deaths every year. That basically equals one in every four deaths in this country.

Every thirty-six seconds someone in America dies from heart disease. That means in the time it took you to read this paragraph, someone's mother, son, or grandfather died from a disease they likely could have prevented.

We often think of overweight middle-aged men dropping dead from heart attacks, but heart disease is also the number one killer of women in America. Especially African American women. According to the American Heart Association (AHA), almost fifty thousand African American women die from heart disease every year. Many more are walking around with a ticking time bomb in their chests but don't even know it. The AHA notes that 49 percent of African American women over the age of twenty have heart disease but only one in five believe that they are personally at risk. Many find out about their condition only after they've already been debilitated by high blood pressure or stroke.

Heart disease is not only crippling people but our economy as well. America is made up of only 5 percent of the global population, yet every year American hospitals perform over half of the angioplasties and bypass procedures in the entire world. The cost for these procedures is almost $50 billion a year. Imagine if we could redirect even just half of that money to education. Or housing. Or job training.

A lot of the money spent "fighting" heart disease is spent on prescription pills. According to the National Center for Health Research, some thirty million Americans currently take drugs like Lipitor, Altoprev, and Crestor to help them stave off the high blood pressure that leads to heart disease.

As astounding as that number is, some say it's still not nearly high enough. In a report for the National Heart, Lung, and Blood Institute, Dr. Lewis Kuller wrote, "All males over 65 years of age, exposed to a traditional Western diet, have cardiovascular disease and should be treated as such."

There are even some health professionals who have recommended that we start putting anticholesterol drugs directly into our water supply. Is this what we really want? A country where every male over the age of sixty-five is living with heart disease? Where almost half the people between ages forty and seventy-five need prescription drugs to stay alive? Drugs that come with side effects like nausea, diarrhea, stomach pain, cramps, and weakness. Remember, those drugs don't *cure* heart disease. They don't address what's making people sick and actually fix it. They just keep you alive, not to mention dependent on the pharmaceutical companies that make them.

Average cholesterol levels:
Meat eaters: 210
Vegetarians: 161
Vegans: 133
 —PETA

For executives in the health-care industry or big pharmaceutical companies, this system is working pretty well. But for everyone else, it's a mess.

Rather than accepting a half million deaths and *trillions* of dollars in medical costs each year (that's right—treating heart disease costs us billions of dollars each year and is expected to cost us over a trillion dollars by 2030), wouldn't it make a lot more sense to change our lifestyles? To give up the products that are killing and crippling us and to replace them with foods that actually make us healthier?

To a growing number of doctors, the answer is a resounding *yes*. One of them shouting it the loudest is a surgeon named Dr. Caldwell

Esselstyn, the author of the best-seller *Prevent and Reverse Heart Disease*. Esselstyn first became interested in heart disease while working at the world-renowned Cleveland Clinic. Frustrated by the sense that he was only treating the symptoms of the diseases he encountered, he began researching what was making Americans so sick, especially with heart disease. "You know what happens when you start to have heart trouble—you have to get put on medication," he says, explaining why he was frustrated by the medical community's traditional approach to the disease. "You undergo numerous surgeries. You develop chest pains called angina, it gets so bad you can't even lie down, you need to sleep sitting up. Most men lose their sexual potency. And that's if you're lucky. If you're unlucky, like millions are, you die."

Esslestyn was determined to find a better way to treat people than just giving them a pill or cutting open their chests. His research showed him there were certain communities around the world—in central Africa, the highlands of Papua New Guinea, and some regions in Mexico—that had almost no incidents of heart disease. When he looked into the traditional diets of those regions, he saw they contained almost no animal products. Heart disease, Esslestyn deduced, must be linked to the prevalence of animal products in the Western diet.

He then convinced the cardiology department at the Cleveland Clinic to let him run a trial program in which he would work with patients who had been diagnosed with severe heart disease and who had already undergone surgery and been told that there was nothing else conventional medicine could do for them. "The worst of the worst," as Esselstyn put it. They had already been given what amounted to death sentences, but Esselstyn was convinced if he put these patients on a plant-based diet, he could not only stop but also reverse their heart disease.

The rules of his diet were pretty simple: Patients couldn't eat anything with a mother or a face. That meant zero meat and fish, and also no dairy products. Since his patients were also in the late stages of heart disease, Esselstyn also added no avocado or oils (olive oil, canola oil, etc.) to the list.

Esselstyn encouraged his patients to eat as many vegetables as possible, especially leafy greens like spinach, kale, chard, collard greens, and bok choy. They could also eat all the whole grains, legumes, and lentils they wanted, as well as fruits.

Within a year, almost all of Esselstyn's patients saw their heart disease improve. Even one of his fellow surgeons at the Cleveland Clinic, who had suffered a major heart attack and been told that he probably wouldn't live past middle age, saw positive changes.

"In fully compliant patients, we have seen angina disappear in a few weeks and abnormal stress test results return to normal," says Esselstyn, adding that there's no need to wait until you have heart disease to switch to a plant-based diet. "The dietary changes that have helped my patients over the past twenty years can help you too. They can actually make you immune to heart attacks."

Probably the most famous person who's beaten heart disease by switching to a plant-based diet is President Bill Clinton. Since his days as governor of Arkansas, he wasn't exactly a poster boy for healthy eating. He pretty much wore his love for hamburgers, hot dogs, and junk food as a badge of honor.

All that meat and grease finally caught up to President Clinton after he left the White House, when doctors checked his heart and discovered he had advanced heart disease. In 2004 he underwent a quadruple bypass surgery, which the doctors assured him would fix the problem. Yet six years later, President Clinton found himself going under the knife again, this time to have two stents inserted into a blocked vein.

President Clinton had started eating healthier and taking blood pressure medication after his first surgery, so he wanted to know why his heart had failed him again. His condition, claimed his doctors, was a result of genetics. He was told he was an "unlucky" person with a "bad heart."

But if we've learned anything about President Clinton over the years, it's that even if he seems to be in a really bad spot he'll figure a way out of it. Fighting heart disease was no different.

Refusing to accept his unlucky diagnosis, one of the first things President Clinton did was read Esselstyn's book. Then he read *The China Study: The Most Comprehensive Study of Nutrition Ever Conducted and the Startling Implications for Diet, Weight Loss, and Long-Term Health* by T. Colin Campbell, which also argues that giving up animal products can help beat heart disease and cancer (more on that book shortly).

Finally, President Clinton got a very direct e-mail from his longtime friend Dr. Dean Ornish of the Preventive Medicine Research Institute in California. In the e-mail, Ornish told the president to stop listening to the doctors who were blaming genetics for his condition. "The friends that mean the most to me are the ones that tell me what I need to hear, not what I want to hear," wrote Ornish, adding that Clinton's best chance to beat heart disease was to adopt a plant-based diet. "And you need to know that your genes are not your fate. And I say this not to blame you, but to empower you."

Thankfully, President Clinton heard Ornish's message and decided to give up animal products (as well as oils because of the advanced stage of his disease) for good.

> "I was lucky that I didn't die.... I don't want it to happen again."
> —Bill Clinton

In a short time, Clinton lost almost twenty-five pounds and saw his energy dramatically improve. Most important, tests showed that his heart disease was in reverse. "I did all this research and I saw that 82 percent of the people since 1986 who have gone on a plant-based [diet], no dairy, no meat of any kind, no chicken or turkey . . . have begun to heal themselves," the president told CNN. "Their arterial blockage cleans up, the calcium deposit around their heart breaks up."

The guy who literally used to jog to McDonald's for a Big Mac now testifies that giving up meat has saved his life. "I went on essentially a plant-based diet. I live on beans, legumes, vegetables, fruits. I drink almond milk mixed with fruit and a protein powder [every morning]. It changed my whole metabolism. And I got back to basically what I weighed in high school."

President Clinton might be the highest-profile example, but his situation is the same one that tens of millions of Americans face every year.

If you've gotten an "unlucky" diagnosis or are related to someone who has been told that the only way to treat heart disease is to have a bypass or get stents stuck in veins, please know that there is another way.

There's no need to join the forty-three million people living in the shadow of heart disease. You have it within your power to make a different choice. What Dean Ornish told President Bill Clinton applies to you too: Your genes are *not* your fate.

CANCER

> *"Research finds that people who eat a diet rich in animal protein carry similar cancer risk to those who smoke twenty cigarettes each day."* —THE DAILY TELEGRAPH

I just mentioned T. Colin Campbell's book *The China Study*, which makes the case that the Western diet contributes to cancer as well as to heart disease.

Campbell took an unlikely path to promoting veganism. Like Esselstyn, he grew up on a dairy farm and believed firmly in the value of drinking milk and eating meat. As a young nutritionist, Campbell's job was helping find new ways to bring high-quality animal protein (that is, meat) to malnourished parts of the Third World. But while working in the Philippines, he made a life-changing discovery. Campbell noticed that children in the upper and middle classes, whose parents could afford to feed them lots of meat, were starting to develop high rates of liver cancer. Among the poor kids Campbell was working with, whose families couldn't afford meat, the incidents of liver cancer were much lower.

Intrigued, Campbell started investigating whether there was a link between eating meat and cancer. Like Esselstyn, he soon recognized that throughout the world there were cultures where there was an unmistakable link between low animal consumption and low cancer rates. After focusing his research on such communities in rural China and Taiwan, he learned about an incredible study the Chinese government had undertaken during the 1970s.

In 1974, the Chinese Prime Minister Zhou Enlai was diagnosed with terminal bladder cancer. Before he died, he directed the government to undertake the most comprehensive cancer study in history, with scientists and researchers tracking almost every reported cancer death in the country over the next ten years.

Campbell was able to gain access to the results of the study, known as the Cancer Atlas. The study showed that throughout China there were higher incidents of cancer in distinct regions throughout the country—what researchers called "cancer clusters." Campbell wanted to know why, so he and Chinese scientist Dr. Junshi Chen embarked on what they called the China Study.

After years of research and analysis, what Campbell and Chen determined was there was a direct link between people's diets and the rate at which they developed cancer. They found that in rural areas where meat was a very small part of people's diets, used almost exclusively for seasoning, there were very low levels of breast, liver, and colorectal cancers.

But in the urban areas, which were quickly beginning to adopt a meat- and dairy-heavy Western diet, incidents of those cancers had begun to rise steadily. The findings were very similar to the connection between meat and liver cancer Campbell had seen in the Philippines.

After years of research, the doctors determined that there was a direct link between meat and cancer. As Chen put it, "The major message from the China Study is a plant-food-based diet, mainly cereal grains, vegetables, and fruit, and very little animal food, is always associated with lower mortality of certain cancers, stroke, and coronary heart disease."

To appreciate the China Study's findings, it helps to understand how cancer actually works. When a lot of people hear the term *cancer*, they think it means you grow a tumor, get sick, and then die. That's not incorrect, but it doesn't tell the whole story either.

Each of our bodies is made up of millions of cells that are meant to divide, or split, over time. That way old cells can die off and new ones can replace them. Sometimes, unfortunately, this process doesn't work right. Instead of dying off, the old cells keep on splitting and then multiplying. When this happens, our body creates more cells than it can handle; these mutated cells begin to mass together and form tumors, which is the stage of the disease that most of us recognize.

The question is, why do some people's cells divide normally, while others begin to mutate into tumors? Campbell's answer was that the enzymes and hormones found in meat created inflammation and high acid levels in people's bodies. It's a climate that cancer is believed to thrive in.

Conversely, Campbell determined that people who ate plant-based diets had less acidic body chemistry. As a result, their cells tended to split normally rather than mutate. For Campbell, the link between animal products and cancer was clear. Switching to and from an animal-based and a plant-based diet was, he said, like "turning the cancer switch on and off."

When Campbell released the findings in *The China Study*, it was hailed as a breakthrough that could potentially save millions of lives. "[These] findings from the most comprehensive large study ever undertaken of the relationship between diet and the risk of developing disease are challenging much of American dietary dogma," wrote the *New York Times*. The American Institute for Cancer Research (AICR) also supported Campbell's findings, saying, "This increased awareness of the importance of plant-based eating is something all of us at AICR welcome."

While *The China Study* received well-deserved praise, Campbell wasn't the only researcher coming to the same conclusion about the link between meat and cancer.

According to the Physicians Committee for Responsible Medicine, "Colorectal cancer is the second most common cancer worldwide with an estimated 80 percent of cases attributable to diet. Previous research indicates that individuals who regularly eat processed or red meat are up to 50 percent more likely to develop colon cancer than individuals who avoid these foods altogether."

Ornish, who encouraged President Clinton to switch to a plant-based diet, has also found that giving up animal products can help you beat cancer. He studied a group of men with prostate cancer and found that those who stopped eating meat and switched to a plant-based diet not only saw their prostate-specific antigen (a blood test that shows the likely presence of cancer cells) stop growing but actually begin to go down. According to Ornish, it was strong evidence that going vegan can not only stop the spread of cancer but actually reverse it.

THE MILK MYTH

> *"Our bodies just weren't made to digest milk on a regular basis. Instead, most scientists agree that it's better for us to get calcium, potassium, protein, and fats from other food sources, like whole plant foods—vegetables, fruits, beans, whole grains, nuts, seeds, and seaweed."*
>
> —DR. MARK HYMAN

I've been talking a lot about the dangers associated with eating meat, but there's also growing evidence of a strong link between dairy and several kinds of health issues, including deadly cancers.

This is why we have to block out the "Milk Does a Body Good" propaganda we've been exposed to all our lives and begin to understand that dairy is actually doing our bodies a lot of *bad*.

To be fair, cow's milk is good for one animal: a calf.

That's about it.

Notice I said *calf*, not even cow. Because what does a cow drink?

Just water.

Not milk.

Think about that: If even *cows* don't drink their milk past infancy, why are so many Americans convinced that it's an essential part of their adult diets? Because our government has told us so. Or more specifically, the USDA has.

According to the USDA, Americans should consume on average at least three cups of milk a day in order to get the daily recommended calcium levels: 1,000 milligrams for people aged eight to fifty and 1,200 milligrams for people fifty years and older. Calcium is believed to help strengthen your bones and prevent fractures.

The USDA has even managed to work dairy into its MyPlate program. An alleged upgrade from the Food Pyramid many of us grew up with, MyPlate is supposed to show Americans what a nutritious dinner plate should look like: roughly equal parts vegetables, fruit, grains, and proteins, with a circle (looking suspiciously like a glass) marked "dairy" next to the plate. Though it's not stated outright, the message of MyPlate is clear: Drink a glass of milk with every meal.

Why is our government suggesting that drinking milk with every meal is a good idea? Because that's what leading doctors have recommended? Of course not!

This is what the doctors at the Harvard School of Public Health have to say about our government pushing the dairy agenda: "MyPlate recommends dairy at every meal, even though there is little if any evidence that high dairy intakes protect against osteoporosis, and there is considerable evidence that too high intakes can be harmful."

Your government isn't promoting dairy because it's good for you; it's promoting it because that's what the dairy lobbyists want. "The USDA is beholden to agriculture," says Susan Levin of the Physicians Committee for Responsible Medicine. "As long as the USDA is in charge of the guidelines, you're going to see them sidestepping good nutrition advice."

> "The guidelines' recommendation to increase the intake of low-fat milk and dairy products seems to reflect the interests of the powerful dairy industry more so than the latest science. There is little, if any, evidence that eating dairy prevents osteoporosis or fractures, and there is considerable evidence that high dairy product consumption is associated with increased risk of fatal prostate and maybe ovarian cancers."
> —Harvard School of Public Health

In the U.K., where the U.S. dairy lobby can't spend any of their budget of hundreds of millions of dollars, scientists say the whole calcium and cow's milk connection is BS. In fact, British researchers say drinking multiple glasses of milk actually makes it *more* likely that you'll suffer a fracture. Even worse, a U.K. study found that people who drank three glasses or more of milk every day were twice as likely to die an early death than those who drank less than one glass per day.

Despite the efforts of the dairy lobby, many highly respected scientists in this country are finally speaking out on the dangers of dairy. Take Dr. Walter Willett of the Department of Nutrition at the Harvard School of Public Health. Despite being a descendant of five generations of dairy farmers (notice a trend here?), Willett has become one of the most vocal critics of the USDA's dairy recommendations. To be clear, Willett isn't some crank doctor on the fringes of the medical world with an ax to grind. This guy is the real deal. The *Boston Globe* calls him "the single-most-cited nutritionist in the world" and notes that among the country's medical elite, "he's Dr. Oz."

So what does one of the nation's top nutritionists, working at one of its top universities, have to say about the USDA's claim we should be drinking more milk? "There is not a single bit of evidence to support that people who drink three servings of milk a day have better health."

As Willett sees it, we've basically been tricked into believing that dairy is a necessary element in our diets. "Humans have no nutritional requirement for animal milk, a relatively recent addition to our diet," he wrote in a recent study. "Anatomically modern humans presumably achieved adequate nutrition for a millennia before domestication of dairy animals, and many populations throughout the world today consume little or no milk for biological reasons (lactase deficiency), lack of availability, or cultural preferences. Adequate dietary calcium for bone health, often cited as the primary rationale for high intakes of milk, can be obtained from many other sources. . . . Throughout the world, bone-fracture rates tend to be lower in countries that do not consume milk compared to those that do."

In layman's terms, we don't need to drink milk. Plus, people who don't drink it are usually healthier than those who do.

Period.

No matter how many celebrities with milk mustaches might say otherwise.

(And by the way, what sort of diet does the country's top

nutritionist—the man who has probably spent more time studying the effects of food on health than anyone else—eat? A meat- and dairy-free diet, of course.)

You probably consume much more dairy than you even realize. You might not drink three cups of milk a day, but all that half-and-half in your coffee, mozzarella on your pizzas, yogurts after lunch, and cheese on your hamburger add up. The average American ends up consuming 607 pounds of milk, cheese, and dairy products every year. That's a lot of dairy clogging up your system!

This is why people who give up dairy often see their allergy problems go away. It will also help with irritable bowel syndrome and digestive problems. I have a lot of friends who say their issues with chronic sinus and ear infection disappeared after they gave up dairy. Almost everyone I know who has gone dairy free has noticed an uptick in their energy levels too.

The biggest health advantage from giving up milk is decreasing your odds of developing several kinds of cancer, including prostate. In an open letter to the medical profession, Willett said, "Consumption of more than two glasses of milk per day was associated with almost twice the risk of advanced and metastatic prostate cancer."

The Harvard School of Public Health, where Willett works, also oversaw a study that charted the health of a group of nurses over a twenty-year period. The study found that nurses who drank one or more glasses of skim or low-fat milk had a 69 percent increase in ovarian cancer over women who rarely or never drank milk. The study also found nurses who ate yogurt five or more times a week had almost double the ovarian cancer rates of nurses who never ate yogurt.

Another study, this one run by the Iowa Women's Health Study, found that postmenopausal women who consumed more than one glass of skim milk a day had a 73 percent greater risk of ovarian cancer than women who didn't drink milk.

Scientists in Sweden decided to explore whether there was a link between countries with high rates of both ovarian cancer and milk consumption. After following more than sixty thousand women for almost fifteen years, researchers found that women who drank more than one glass of milk a day had double the risk of the most deadly forms of ovarian cancer.

Every year, twenty-seven thousand men die from prostate cancer in the United States and fifteen thousand women are lost to ovarian cancer. New research is making it clear that a lot of those deaths could be avoided by simply giving up dairy. Is milk in your coffee or cheese on your pizza really worth the risk?

OBESITY, METABOLIC SYNDROME, AND DIABETES

> *"Red-meat consumption is already linked to higher levels of colorectal cancer and cardiovascular disease (atherosclerosis, heart disease, and stroke). Now researchers from Harvard School of Public Health (HSPH) have added an increased risk of type 2 (adult onset) diabetes to that list."*
>
> —*HARVARD MAGAZINE*

I needed to focus on heart disease and cancer because so many of us are affected by, or at least aware of, them. But it needs to be pointed out that they are far from being the only conditions linked to eating animal products.

Take metabolic syndrome. You might not be familiar with metabolic syndrome, but between 20 and 25 percent of adult Americans suffer from it. The Mayo Clinic describes it as "a cluster of conditions—increased blood pressure, a high blood sugar level, excess body fat around the waist, and abnormal cholesterol levels—that occur together, increasing your risk of heart disease, stroke, and diabetes."

Even if you don't feel out of shape, if you eat the Standard American Diet, you are greatly at risk for metabolic syndrome. Especially if you're African American, Hispanic, Asian, or Native American. I have a friend who is thin and follows a very active lifestyle. But his job has him on the road most of the day, and he almost exclusively ate burgers from fast-food joints. He was astonished when he failed a routine blood sugar test and was diagnosed with prediabetes and metabolic syndrome.

You're probably more familiar with the term *obesity*, which is another condition linked to animal products. We tend to think of it as a term that applies only to "really fat" people, but that's not the case. According to the CDC, almost 35 percent of the American population, or close to seventy-eight million people, are clinically obese. In African Americans, that number is even higher, at almost 48 percent. That means out of every three people reading the book, one of you is obese. And if you're African American, that likelihood shoots up to one out of every two.

Of course, I don't need to quote studies to let you know we have an obesity problem in the United States—you see the evidence every time you walk outside. Or maybe even just look in the mirror.

The effects of obesity are wide ranging. Emotionally, it makes you feel bad about yourself. No one feels good buying an extra-large shirt so they can hide their gut or walking around in sweatpants all the time because their jeans don't fit anymore. Just as no one likes having to tilt their head or try to look serious by resting their chin in their hand every time they pose for a picture because they're embarrassed by their double chin.

Obesity and metabolic syndrome are also becoming major problems for young people. According to the CDC, childhood obesity has more than doubled in children and quadrupled in adolescents in the last thirty years. In 1980, 7 percent of American children were obese. In 2012, that number was up to 18 percent. In 1980, just 5 percent of adolescents were obese, though that number was up to 21 percent in 2012. Overall in 2012, more than one-third of all American young people were either overweight or obese.

As a parent, those numbers are really troubling. The idea of millions of young people feeling fat and uncomfortable is really sad to me.

But again, let's forget about the emotional toll. The bigger issue is if this trend is allowed to continue unchecked, we are literally setting our younger generations up for an early death. Out of those 21 percent of young people who are currently obese, 70 percent of them already have one risk factor of cardiovascular disease. Almost 40 percent have two. These kids are basically heart attacks waiting to happen because of their diets. That's heartbreaking.

But one of the worst dangers of childhood obesity is that it often leads to diabetes, which is becoming a serious epidemic in this country. According to the Harvard School of Public Health, there is a direct link between eating red meat and the disease, especially type 2 diabetes. The study found the best way to prevent diabetes is to replace red meat in a person's diet with whole grains and nuts. "This is [strong] evidence that red meat consumption contributes to an increased risk of diabetes," said the study's author, Frank Hu of Harvard.

Researchers in Singapore recently came to a similar conclusion, writing that giving up red meat cuts down on the chances of developing type 2 diabetes by almost half. "There is no need to have more red meat on your plate," said researcher An Pan of the National University of Singapore. "It increases the risk of diabetes."

Sadly, not nearly enough Americans have gotten the message. Currently twenty-five million people, over 8 percent of our population, suffer from some form of diabetes. That's twice the rate of the rest of the world.

The numbers are getting worse among young people. A new study published in the *Journal of the American Medical Association* found that, between 2000 and 2009, diabetes in kids has increased dramatically. Type 1 diabetes, which is considered an autoimmune disease, increased 21 percent during that period.

Cases of type 2 diabetes, which used to be known as "adult diabetes," are up 30 percent among young people. "It's frightening to see how severe this metabolic disease is in children," Dr. David Nathan, the director of the Diabetes Clinical Center at Massachusetts General Hospital, told the *New York Times*. "It's really got a hold on them, and it's hard to turn around." Noting that childhood diabetes leads to increased risk of heart disease, eye problems, nerve damage, amputations, and kidney failure as adults, Nathan said, "I fear these children are going to become sick earlier in their lives than we've ever seen before."

To make matters worse, many young people with diabetes aren't receiving proper medical care. According to a CDC study, one in five often go over six months without being monitored by a doctor, which is basically the same thing as playing Russian roulette with their health. Dr. Gerald Bernstein, who runs the diabetes program at Mount Sinai Beth Israel in New York City, says that as bad as they are, the current statistics on diabetes represent only the "tip of the iceberg" because "underneath there are millions of people with pre-diabetes, most of whom are not diagnosed." Unless something is done, he says, we're going to pay dearly as a society. "If you don't prevent the diseases, there will be serious medical and economic consequences."

Is this an America you want to live in? Where a large part of our adult population is obese? Where our children are developing diabetes at an alarming rate? Where young people are on course to die before they ever get to grow old?

If your answer is no, then I've got some good news. We can turn this situation around by simply making smarter choices with our food—by eating more vegetables and eliminating animal products. Because, yes, studies have shown that a plant-based diet will not only help prevent but also reverse both obesity and diabetes.

The vast majority of people who go vegan lose weight, in most cases over twenty pounds. The reason I can't say everyone is because you can still go vegan and make poor food choices. If you give up meat, but eat a ton of french fries, potato chips, cereals, white breads, and processed foods and wash them all down with soda, you can still be at risk for obesity and diabetes. And if you don't commit to making exercise a steady part of your lifestyle, even if you stay away from the processed foods, your weight still probably won't change that much either.

But if you stay away from the chips and other processed foods, get plenty of exercise, and really build your diet around whole plant food, the weight is going to come off too. Even better, it'll stay off. According to PETA, going vegetarian is the only diet that's scientifically proven not only to help you lose but to keep your weight off for over a year.

This is why if you or someone you know is dealing with diabetes, please talk to a doctor about going on a plant-based diet. And if the doctor you talk to doesn't see the benefit in that, then go find another doctor or request a referral to see a nutritionist. There's just too much evidence out there that supports the impact giving up animal products has on both obesity and diabetes to just accept that you have to live— or die—with those conditions.

ANTIBIOTICS

> *"Farm animals get 80 percent of antibiotics sold in the United States."* —WIRED

While we're on the subject of young people's health, I want to touch on the connection between antibiotics and eating animals. If you're a parent, you're probably aware that over the last decade or so doctors have become very concerned about the dangers posed by overexposure to antibiotics.

Back in the day, antibiotics were like aspirin—doctors would prescribe them for almost anything. Your daughter has an ear infection? Give her an antibiotic. Your son has a sinus infection? Let's try an antibiotic.

Today, those attitudes have changed dramatically. We know the more antibiotics someone takes, the more resistance they'll build up to them, so that when you really need antibiotics to kick in, they might not work.

There's a growing fear that antibiotic-resistant "superbugs" will be one of the biggest crises humanity faces going forward. One new study even says superbugs could kill three hundred million people by 2050 unless we slow down our intake of antibiotics and learn to use them more wisely. MRSA, which is an antibiotic-resistant staph infection, already kills ninety thousand Americans every year, more than we lost to AIDS.

Yet even as doctors become more selective with how they prescribe antibiotics, as a society we're not doing enough to address the biggest antibiotic consumers out there. And it's not kids with sore throats or adults with sinus infections.

It's factory farm animals.

The animals we eat are themselves consuming close to *thirty million pounds* of antibiotics every year.

That takes place for a couple of reasons: The first is that many factory farmers feed their animals proactively to keep them "healthy." A farmer with thirty thousand chickens can't check each bird to see if it's getting sick. Instead he just feeds all those birds antibiotics every day figuring that the sick ones will get the medicine they need.

Factory farmers also like antibiotics because they make animals gain weight faster. The more the animals weigh when they're killed, the more the factory farms get paid. Plus, Americans don't like lean meat. We like our meat fatty, or "marbled," as it's called in the industry. Giving animals antibiotics helps ensure they'll get nice and fat before they're killed.

Tellingly, there's no system that forces farmers to be selective with how they use antibiotics. If you or I needed antibiotics, we'd have to go to a doctor and get a prescription. The doctor would instruct us how much to take and for how long.

But if you owned a big chicken farm and you wanted to give your birds thirty thousand pounds of antibiotics, there would be no need to go to a veterinarian for a prescription. The FDA recently suggested farmers do so, but ultimately that decision is "voluntary." You could go to a feed store and buy however much you want. It's insane that drugs we regulate so closely in human consumption are essentially unregulated when it comes to the animals we eat.

Antibiotics aren't the only drugs you're unwittingly eating either. Did you know that chickens are fed Prozac? That's right, a study of commercial chicken meat by Johns Hopkins University found that many of the birds had been given Prozac, in addition to painkillers, antibiotics, and allergy medication. Why Prozac? Because without an antidepressant, they might die from stress. That's how terrible the conditions they live in are.

It's crazy that so many people now go out of their way to make sure they doesn't abuse antibiotics or needlessly take drugs like Prozac, but then unwittingly ingest those very same drugs every day via the meat they eat. It might not be pleasant to think about, but you have to accept that every time your kid has a piece of steak or bite of chicken, they are likely consuming antibiotics.

The danger is that, over time, antibiotics won't be as effective on you or your child as they might be on someone who doesn't eat meat.

Your strep throat might take longer to go away. An infection might take longer to heal. When you really need antibiotics to work, like when a superbug develops, a resistance could lead to death.

That might sound dramatic, but remember: You're not just what you eat. You're what you eat eats too. And as long as you're eating the meat from animals that are fed antibiotics every day, you're going to be increasing the chances that you've built up a resistance to those drugs. Drugs that could very well one day mean the difference between sickness and health. Or life and death.

NOT YOUR FATE

> *"When we become more aware of how powerfully our choices in diet and lifestyle affect us—for better and for worse—then we can make different ones."*
>
> —DR. DEAN ORNISH

Sorry if I've been painting a bleak picture in this section. This was supposed to be the *happy* vegan, right? It might seem hard to feel happy thinking about how almost half of our adult population is obese. About how our children are developing diabetes at an alarming rate. About how young people are on course to die before they ever get to grow old.

There is some happy news, however. And it's that we can turn the situation around. Without drugs, shots, or pills. By doing nothing more than cutting out meat and dairy from our diet and eating more vegetables.

Whether you are a former president or a single mother in a housing project, *you* have a very large say over whether or not you will fall victim to these diseases.

Despite what you might be told, there is no pill and no procedure that will help you live longer than simply eating a plant-based diet. Let's be real: If there were, you know President Clinton would have gotten it a long time ago.

Luckily, when it comes to diet, we're all on the same playing field. If you cut out animal products and build your diet around plants, you are giving yourself *much* better odds to not be that one-in-three American who is going to get cancer in their lifetime.

For me, that person was my mother. Every son loves his mother, but my mother and I had an especially close bond. I wasn't an easy child to raise—I was a dreamer with ADD. My constant hustlin' used to drive my parents nuts. But no matter what sort of trouble I'd gotten myself into, my mother always had my back. I've told this story before, but when I was in college I lost all my money trying to promote a rap concert, and most of my family was ready to give up on me. It was my mother who took some money out of a secret stash she kept, gave it to me, and told me to try again. I've never forgotten that love and faith she showed in me in that moment.

So it was very hard for my brothers and me when my mother came down with throat cancer. We made sure she got the best doctors and we would go back to Queens to sit beside her when the chemotherapy made her too weak to get out of bed. Ultimately, there was very little we could do. As a father to two girls, I can't help but sometimes think about what a great presence she would have been in my daughters' lives. The cancer cut that relationship way too short.

If I had known what I know now about the connection between diet and disease, I would have encouraged my mother to switch to a plant-based diet before the cancer showed up in her throat. Just as I would have encouraged my father to make that switch before Alzheimer's disease turned an incredibly dynamic and charismatic man into a shell of his former self. And yes, studies have shown that there is a link between meat and Alzheimer's too.

It's too late for my parents. But it might not be too late for yours. Or your children. Or your friends.

Or you.

GETTING THE MOST OUT OF LIFE

> *"Nothing will benefit human health and increase the chances for survival of life on Earth as much as the evolution to a vegetarian diet."* —ALBERT EINSTEIN

Considering what's at stake, I had to share that information about the links between eating meat and preventable diseases. Depressing or not.

I don't, however, want to create the impression that your main motivation for going vegan should be avoiding an early death.

Instead, one of the best motivations for giving up animal products should be how much more it will help you get the most out of *life*.

Going vegan is going to help you feel incredible physically. I might not be a world-class athlete like the MMA fighters or pro football players I mentioned earlier, but don't sleep on me either. In my twenties and thirties I was round and bloated and felt and looked like crap most of the time. One of the reasons I spent so much time getting high was to distract myself from having to confront how much I'd let my body go.

Today I'm much smaller. I might not have a six-pack, but there's no doubt that I'm in much, much better shape than I've ever been in my life. Whether it's in yoga, on the treadmill, or in the boardroom, I can more than hold my own with the thirty- and even twenty-year-olds. I attribute so much of that vitality to my diet.

My friend the rapper Snoop Dogg commented on this recently when I appeared on his show, *GGN*. "You looking good, you living good, you damn near look like you're going backwards," he told me. "Like you're twentysomething damn years old."

"I'm older than a motherfucker, Snoop," I replied.

"You know *I* know, but you look like you going backwards. Like you age is running that way instead of that way. Is it what you eat?"

"I think it's happiness," I told him, before explaining that eating a compassionate diet is a big part of what makes me happy. "I don't eat any animal products—no meat, dairy, eggs, fish—none of that shit . . . and that helps a lot."

Then I gave Snoop the same rap I'm giving you in this book, explaining why giving up animal products is so important to us as individuals and collectively. Snoop paused and wistfully rubbed his chin. "Damn. Barbecued ribs, filet mignon . . . damn . . . that's hard to give up."

To prove my point that it actually wasn't hard at all, I gave Snoop a Super Italian Meatball Sub (the meatball is made from seitan instead of beef) from Native Foods, a vegan restaurant in Los Angeles. By the end of the episode, Snoop was sold. "That motherfucking meatball good," he said between bites. "Or whatever it is."

Snoop might think I'm looking younger, but it's a different story for a lot of the people in my age group that I grew up with. It pains me to say this, but a lot of them are dying. They need pills just to get through the day. They walk slow, they talk slow, and their brains seem to have started to slow down. A lot of these folks seem like they're on their final run, like they've resigned themselves to their fate.

Maybe Snoop's right, because I feel like I am moving in the opposite direction. I haven't had a cold or felt rundown in close to five years. I have to attribute a lot of that to not eating animals. It only stands to reason that I'd get healthier once I stopped ingesting sickness and sadness on a daily basis.

There are so many who feel like they've been able to reclaim their bodies—and their lives—by giving up animal products. For some, like the boxing great Mike Tyson, it was a step that they credit for saving their lives. After retiring from the ring, Mike fell into the vicious circle of drug and alcohol abuse. He gained a ton of weight and was in really bad shape by the time he hit his forties. "I was so congested from all the drugs and bad cocaine that I could hardly breathe. I had high blood pressure, I had arthritis . . . I was dying," he told Oprah. "Once I became a vegan, all that stuff diminished."

I also know plenty of people who were already living clean and healthy lives but saw giving up animal products as a way to get the most out of the work they were putting into their bodies. A great example is my niece Angela Simmons, who has been a vegetarian since I showed her and her family *Diet for a New America* several years ago. Detaching herself from the abuse of the animals was a big motivation for her, but she was also attracted to the idea that a plant-based diet would give her more energy during her workouts. Once she made the switch, she found that her energy and stamina increased almost at once. Tapping into that new power source, she was able to dedicate herself to an intense schedule of yoga, kickboxing, cross-training, and weight lifting, and has managed to work herself into absolutely incredible shape. I've been so proud to watch her transform from someone who was dealing with the body issues young women face into a completely empowered young woman.

> "I've been vegetarian for four years and I love it. I feel lighter. It's a good feeling."
> —Angela Simmons

That sense of vitality and empowerment isn't going to be limited to only your body when you give up animal products. The mind–body connection that yogis talk about is real. Your body is truly your temple, and when you take care of it, that sense of health and vitality will translate to your outlook on life too.

A recent study published in *Nutrition Journal* found that there is a direct link between having a positive outlook on life and not eating meat. According to the study's authors, the high amounts of fatty acids found in factory farm meat has negative effects on people's moods. "Restricting meat, fish, and poultry improved . . . short-term mood state in modern omnivores," the study concluded.

I'm glad scientists are starting to look into this connection because I can attest from personal experience that it is real. It's really just common sense. Any time you step out of a harmful cycle and into a good one, it's going to make you feel happier about your place in the world.

We accept that this is true for people who step out of a harmful cycle of drug abuse. Or the harmful cycle of a dysfunctional relationship. Or the harmful cycle of crime. Well, it's no different with what you eat. When you let go of the negativity that comes from ingesting death, you are going to feel happier and more upbeat about your relationship with the world.

We always hear about the former drug addict or ex-criminal getting a new lease on life. That same lease is waiting for you. All you have to do is let go of the foods that are not only aging you but killing you too, and start eating a diet that promotes life.

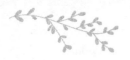

DO IT FOR THE EARTH

"The livestock sector emerges as one of the top two or three most significant contributors to the most serious environmental problems, at every scale from local to global."

—UN REPORT, "LIVESTOCK'S LONG SHADOW"

In the last chapter, I shared compelling reasons to give up meat and dairy for your health.

Now I want to share some facts about why giving up meat and dairy is critical for someone else's health too:

Mother Earth's.

"Livestock production is one of the major causes of the world's most pressing environmental problems, including global warming, land degradation, air and water pollution, and loss of biodiversity."

—UN report, "Livestock Impacts on the Environment"

You're probably aware that even more so than poverty, hunger, overpopulation, and disease, the destruction of the environment is arguably the greatest threat we face collectively as a species. What you might not be aware of, however, is just how large a role the meat and dairy industries play in that destruction.

Which is why after reading this chapter, I hope you'll agree with me that the single best thing you can do to help the environment is to stop eating animal products.

Don't get me wrong—it's great if you go out of your way to lighten your carbon footprint. If you recycle your paper and plastics, please don't stop. Keep using efficient lightbulbs and be sure you don't run your shower any more than you have to. It's wonderful if you take public transportation whenever possible and drive a hybrid when you do have to use a car. You're setting a powerful example.

But none of those well-intentioned steps will match the positive impact you'll have on the environment by simply giving up animal products.

Here's why.

UNDERSTAND THE SCALE

> *"The average person will chomp down on 7,000 animals during their life."* —USA TODAY

Intuitively, you probably know that people consume a lot of meat and dairy in this country. After all, from Queens to Compton, from Houston to Chicago, from Montana to Maine, have you ever been to a grocery store anywhere that wasn't stocked with chicken, pork, and beef? That didn't carry milk and cheese? Of course not. No matter what the region or season, meat and dairy are always available.

But have you ever thought about what it actually means to be able to go into *any* supermarket in the country and buy a hamburger? Have you considered just how many farm animals we need to raise in order for their meat to be available everywhere, every day of the year?

Probably not.

So let's look at some of the numbers.

According to the USDA, in 2012 10.2 *billion* animals were raised and killed for food in the United States. A staggering number when you consider that "only" 314 million people lived in the country that year.

It's not surprising that those 10-plus billion animals are taking up a lot of space. A study published by the USDA found that 80 percent of agricultural land in this country is used either to raise animals or to grow the crops—corn, grain, oats, and so on—to feed them. That's equal to almost half the total landmass of the lower forty-eight states.

Across the globe, the numbers are just as staggering. According to the United Nations, the land used for grazing "occupies 26 percent of the Earth's terrestrial surface, while feed-crop production requires about a third of all arable land."

The UN also estimates that worldwide 65 billion land animals are killed every year for food (we won't even mention the billions, possibly even trillions, of marine animals killed every year). Scientists says that unless we slow down the global demand for meat, in the next few decades that number could rise to 120 billion land animals killed every year.

Take a second and really let those numbers sink in:

- 65 billion animals killed every year.
- 65 billion animals that needed space to live.
- 65 billion animals that needed food to eat.
- 65 billion animals that needed water to drink.
- 65 billion animals that pissed and shat every day.

If you really consider what it means to house, feed, and dispose of the waste of 65 billion animals, then you'll have to admit that we are testing Mother Nature like we never have before. You can try to justify the situation by saying, "Hey, this is just how people eat," but history says otherwise. We've been producing meat on this scale for only the last fifty years, which in the scope of human history is barely the blink of an eye. Even only one hundred years ago, Americans were eating 9.8 billion pounds of meat a year, compared with the 52 billion pounds we're eating today. That means our meat consumption has more than quadrupled in less than a century.

This is not a sustainable way of life. Unless more and more people make the choice to give up meat, we will be buttressing up a system that in the not too distant future is going to come crashing down on us.

> "If the current world population at 7 billion were to adopt North America's meat-based diet, it would require four planet earths to support this demand."
>
> —*Vancouver Sun*

If we want to live in a world where global warming hasn't made conditions unlivable, we have to break our addiction to meat. If we want to live in a world where the rivers aren't polluted, we have to break our addiction to meat. If we want to live in a world where there's enough water for us to share, we have to break our addiction to meat.

There is no other choice.

CLIMATE CHANGE

> *"If we're honest, less meat is also good for the health, and would also at the same time reduce emissions of greenhouse gases."*
>
> —DR. RAJENDRA PACHAURI, HEAD OF THE UN
> INTERGOVERNMENTAL PANEL ON CLIMATE CHANGE

Back in the early 1990s I can remember bumping into a friend who had just come from a lecture by the comedian and social activist Dick Gregory.

"Ah, that man is crazy," my friend told me after I asked how the lecture was. "He was up there talking about how cows' farts are what's creating the hole in the ozone layer."

We both laughed—after all, the idea of cow farts poking a hole in the sky *is* pretty funny—and dismissed Dick's theory as a wild conspiracy. All these years later, however, it's become clear that Dick was right and the joke was actually on us.

The evidence is now irrefutable that the methane produced by cows is one of the leading causes of greenhouse gasses. Those are the harmful gases that float to the top of the earth's atmosphere and collect heat, creating a greenhouse-like condition on earth that eventually results in global warming.

Here's why cows produce so much methane: Cows are designed to eat grass. That grass goes into one of the cow's four different stomachs and is then regurgitated back up as "cud," which the cow chews and digests all over again. All that chewing, regurgitating, and digesting creates an unusually large amount of methane in their gut, gas that has to go somewhere. Most of it is released when a cow burps or poops (only a small bit actually comes from farts—Dick was wrong about that), which, if you've ever been around cows, you know that they do constantly.

According to the Environmental Protection Agency (EPA), a single cow belches out between 66 to 132 gallons of methane a day. (A car, by comparison, holds only about 16 gallons of gas in its tank.) That means billions of gallons of methane are being burped out every day and floating directly into the atmosphere. Once it's up there, the methane is very effective at trapping heat, even more so than carbon dioxide, the gas that most people associate with global warming.

Scientists at NASA say that methane is actually twenty-five times more potent as a greenhouse gas than is CO_2.

Because methane is so effective at trapping heat, scientists at the UN now believe that gasses produced by animal agriculture are responsible for 18 percent of all greenhouse gas emissions. Conversely, the combined fossil fuels (coal, gas, oil, etc.) used to power the automobile, train, and airline industries account for only 13 percent of greenhouse gas emissions. That means by eating beef, you're actually contributing to global warming more than you are by driving cars, riding trains, or flying in planes.

By giving up meat, you'd be helping not only to cut down on but actually to reverse global warming. When CO_2 is emitted into the air via fossil fuels like coal and gas, it stays in the atmosphere for almost a century. Methane, on the other hand, cycles out of the environment after just eight years. "If you reduce the amount of methane emissions, the level in the atmosphere goes down very quickly, as in decades," Berkeley professor Kirk Smith says in *Cowspiracy*. "As opposed to CO_2, if you reduce the emissions to the atmosphere, you won't really see a signal in the atmosphere for a hundred years or so."

Animal agriculture also contributes to global warming by helping destroy the Amazon rain forest. The rain forest performs several critical functions in our ecosystem: Its trees and plants give us 20 percent of the oxygen we breathe on earth as well as 60 percent of all our fresh water. It also does an excellent job protecting the ozone layer by absorbing greenhouse gasses (like the methane) before they reach the atmosphere. It would likely be catastrophic if we lost the Amazon rain forest, but that's exactly what's happening.

Despite our ecological reliance on the trees (to say nothing of the millions of animal species that live in them), the rain forest is being cut down at an alarming rate. Every second, an acre of trees is cleared. That equals an area larger than the size of Florida being lost every year. What are most of these trees being cleared for? You guessed it, raising animals. Especially cattle. Brazil has the largest commercial cattle herd in the world and between 1996 and 2006 an area the size of Portugal was carved out of the rain forest to create land for them to graze on. "The driving force behind all of this is animal agriculture," says Dr. Oppenlander from *Cowspiracy*. "Ninety-one percent of the rain forest that's been destroyed has been due to raising livestock."

WASTING WATER

> *"Farm animals use more than half the water consumed in the United States."*
>
> —JOHN ROBBINS, *THE FOOD REVOLUTION*

A couple of years ago I moved to Los Angeles and bought a beautiful house in the Hollywood Hills. One of the things that attracted me to the house was that it has a small (at least by L.A. standards) backyard pool surrounded by hedges, flowers, and a lemon tree. I love to sit out there and meditate. It's like my own little Garden of Eden.

Throughout the city, people have created similar little Gardens of Eden for themselves—houses with pools, hedges, flowers, and mani-cured lawns. If you drive through neighborhoods like the Hills, or Beverly Hills, or Brentwood early in the morning, you'll see armies of

Mexican workers arriving to clean the pools and landscape the yards and gardens.

There's just one problem (outside of the fact that those workers have very little rights, are underpaid, and are largely ignored by the rest of the city—but that's a subject for another book): All those gardens, pools, and lawns require water to be maintained. And water is something that Los Angeles doesn't have nearly enough of.

It can be easy to forget, but the city was built on a desert and doesn't possess its own water supply. It has to pipe it in from northern California or the Colorado River Basin. I'm writing this in the summer of 2015, and water levels in those areas get dangerously low. The drought of 2014 was deemed the worst one in 150 years, and experts are worried that this summer could be even worse. As a result, the state has ordered emergency measures to slash water usage in urban areas by 25 percent. People all over California are scrambling to cut back on the amount of water they use by taking shorter showers, replacing grass with rock and shrubs in their landscaping, and using more water-efficient appliances. Workers are being sent out to repair leaky sprinklers and water mains.

> "Californians use 1,500 gallons of water per person per day. Close to half is associated with meat and dairy products."
> —Pacific Institute, "California's Water Imprint"

We'll probably make it through the drought this summer, but experts say we might not be so lucky next time. You might not be either.

While droughts so far have affected only areas of the West and Southwest, if we don't find a way to conserve water, the rest of the country might soon be in the same situation as California. "All Around the U.S., Risks of a Water Crisis Are Much Bigger Than People Realize" was the title of a 2013 *Business Insider* article. The piece quoted a study by the Columbia University Water Center, which said that several major metropolitan areas, including New York City and Washington, D.C., as well as large parts of the Great Plains, are all expected to face major water shortages in the near future. While below-average rainfall is part of the problem, the study noted the bigger issue is that water usage in the country has gone up 127 percent since 1950. Maybe that's why a recent study by the firm Ernst & Young found that 76 percent of corporate leaders think that water is our nation's top security risk.

That's true for so many countries around the globe. From Saudi Arabia to India to China, governments are jockeying to control the water resources in their regions because they know in a few years there just won't be enough to go around.

Many experts predict that the wars of the next century won't be waged over land or oil but over water. "I think the risk of conflicts over water is growing—not shrinking—because of increased competition, because of bad management, and, ultimately, because of the impacts of climate change," Peter Gleick of the Pacific Institute tells the U.K.'s *Guardian*.

To avoid a future where we're scrounging for and fighting over water, we have to reassess how we use it today. We can cut back on showers and fix leaky sprinklers, but those are only going to be small steps toward addressing the larger problem. That's because the majority of the water we consume in this country is used for raising farm animals, not watering our lawns or filling up our pools.

According to the USDA, private homes represent about 5 percent of the water consumed in the United States. Animal agriculture, on the hand, represents 55 percent of the water we use. That might seem hard to believe, but raising the animals we eat requires a lot of water each year— over fifteen *trillion* gallons, according to a study by the *Oxford Journal*.

You might be saying to yourself, "Sorry, Russell, there's no way cows and pigs are drinking fifteen trillion gallons of water every year." And you'd be right. They're *drinking* only about one trillion gallons a year. But they're also eating massive amounts of grain, corn, soybean, and alfalfa hay, crops that are grown in irrigated fields. When you factor in all the water required to grow those crops, you're looking at another fourteen trillion gallons of water a year going toward the meat that we eat.

> "The water needed to produce 10 pounds of steak is the same as the amount an average household uses in a year."
> —*Diet for a Small Planet*

Every time you eat meat, you are contributing to our water crisis way more than you realize. Say you go to your favorite fast-food joint and order a cheeseburger. According to the PETA, 660 gallons of water were needed to produce that one single burger. If you buy a pound of ground beef, 1,799 gallons of water were needed to produce that single package. "Animals raised for food have to eat as many as 13 pounds of grain to create just one pound of edible flesh," reports PETA.

If you still can't see why the meat industry is responsible for so much water usage, consider this visual: You could literally float a battleship on the amount of water that's needed to raise a single thousand-pound beef cow. Not a rowboat. Or a tugboat. Or even a yacht.

I said a *battleship*.

Then consider that there are almost ninety million cattle being raised for food in this country. Try to picture the amount of water needed to keep ninety million battleships afloat. It's hard to even conceive of.

Dairy and eggs are draining their fair share of water too. About 700 gallons of water go into producing a pound of cheese; 477 gallons of water are needed to produce a pound of eggs. By comparison, a *National Geographic* study found that producing a pound of potatoes requires only 119 gallons of water, a pound of corn needs 108 gallons, and a pound of wheat uses 132 gallons.

> "Cutting back on meat consumption would protect waterways from pollution caused by fertilizer production, runoff from chemical fertilizer and manure, and soil erosion. Of course, producing more fruits, vegetables, beans, and nuts still would require water, but far less than is needed to produce animal products."
>
> —Center for Science in the Public Interest

This is why when we look at ways to improve how we use water, we need to stop thinking only in terms of personal consumption. Again, cutting back on showers and watering your lawn are important, but they are only, no pun intended, tiny drops in the bucket compared to the amount of water that goes toward raising farm animals. You could literally not shower for six months and you would save the same amount of water as you would by not buying a pound of beef.

If you were to cut meat out of your diet, you'd be saving an estimated 162,486 gallons of water each year. That would represent over 50 percent of your annual water consumption.

Imagine if millions of other people went vegan too. Then eventually tens of millions more did the same thing. We'd be saving so much water and sparing ourselves (and our children) so much of the suffering we're bound to face if we keep on dedicating so much of this precious resource to raising animals for their meat.

RUINING OUR RIVERS

> *"The amount of manure generated in the United States at CAFOs and ASOs is estimated to exceed 335 million tons of dry matter per year."* —USDA

I wish I could stop here, but it also needs to be pointed out that the waste created by factory farm animals is absolutely devastating our waterways. If we don't do something about it soon, we're going to be a nation of dead rivers and creeks.

How's it happening? In the simplest terms, the animals we raise for food in this country poop a lot. And much of that poop is ending up in our water.

When I say these farm animals "poop a lot," I mean in massive amounts. A study by the U.S. Senate Committee on Agriculture, Nutrition, and Forestry found that animals produce 1.37 billion *tons* of solid animal waste in the United States each year. That's 130 times more waste than humans produce.

It's no surprise that cows are the biggest offenders when it comes to emptying their bowels. According to the EPA, "the waste produced per day by one dairy cow is equal to 20–40 people." A dairy farm with twenty-five thousand cows creates the same amount of poop each year as a city with a population of four hundred thousand people. That means a medium-size dairy farm is creating more poop each year than Miami. But while there aren't even fifty cities the size of Miami in the United States, according to the EPA there are more than *nine hundred thousand* dairy farms.

Pigs also contribute more than their fair share to this poop parade. A single hog excretes almost eighty pounds of waste per day. According to the CDC, "a feeding operation with 800,000 pigs could produce over 1.6 million tons of waste a year. That amount is one and a half times more than the annual sanitary waste produced by the city of Philadelphia, Pennsylvania."

Of course when the humans in Miami or Philly poop, they do it (we hope) in a toilet. That waste is then carried through pipes to a water treatment plant, where it's decontaminated before it's sent back into local rivers or oceans. Even that process is pretty disgusting when you think about it. But at least the water *is* being treated.

When it comes to all that animal waste, we don't have any plans in place. As the CDC notes, "Though sewage treatment plants are required for human waste, no such treatment facility exists for livestock waste."

> "Contamination from runoff or lagoon leakage can degrade water resources, and can contribute to illness by exposing people to wastes and pathogens in their drinking water. Dust and odors can contribute to respiratory problems in workers and nearby residents."
>
> —Environmental Protection Agency

Back in the day, this wasn't a big problem. Farms had fewer animals and much more land for them to graze on. Farmers would take the waste that their animals produced and turn it into manure, which they would use to fertilize those fields for grazing. It was a very sustainable system—the animals would eat grass and poop. The poop would be turned into fertilizer to grow more grass.

That kind of sustainability, however, is long gone. A farm with ten thousand pigs or a hundred thousand chickens produces much more animal waste than could ever be used to fertilize fields.

So where does all that excess waste go?

Not far.

The waste is mixed with water and then dumped into massive pits—or lagoons, as they're called in the industry—next to the factory farms where the animals are raised. We're not talking about little ponds or pools either. These lagoons are often the size of several football fields, each filled to the brim with a putrid sea of animal pee and poop.

According to the EPA, there are currently 450,000 of these lagoons scattered around the country. They are supposed to be constructed with reinforced walls and embankments so that the toxic waste doesn't leak out, but those precautions aren't always effective. A study by North Carolina State University estimated that 55 percent of the lagoons on hog factory farms have experienced leaks.

Because heavy rains can also cause these lagoons to flood or leak, the CDC has identified waste from factory farms as one of the greatest threats to our nation's waterways. "The agriculture sector [factory farms] is the leading contributor of pollutants to lakes, rivers, and reservoirs. It has been found that states with high concentrations of [factory farms] experience on average 20 to 30 serious water-quality problems per year as a result of manure management problems."

The problem is that once spilled or leaked waste is in the soil, it will eventually make its way as runoff into local streams or creeks, where it wreaks serious damage. Animal waste is very high in nitrate, which is harmful to humans. In 1996, the CDC established a link between spontaneous abortions and high nitrate levels in Indiana drinking-water wells located near feedlots. High nitrate levels in drinking water also lead to methemoglobinemia, or blue baby syndrome, which kills hundreds of infants every year.

Let's also remember that most of those animals are being fed antibiotics, which is present in their waste. When the waste leaks, those antibiotics eventually make their way into rivers, creeks, and ultimately our drinking water. Which in turn makes us even more susceptible to antibiotic-resistant bacteria.

The drugs in animal waste are particularly damaging to fish. In 1995, an eight-acre lagoon on a North Carolina hog farm burst, sending twenty-five million gallons of waste into a local river. Ten million fish were killed and 364,000 acres of coastal wetlands had to be closed for shellfish harvesting. In 2011, a lagoon on an Illinois factory farm burst, sending two hundred thousand gallons of waste into a local creek. Over a hundred thousand fish were killed in that spill.

In the rivers and streams of Maryland and West Virginia, male fish have begun growing ovaries. Scientists believe it's due to the presence of antibiotics and Prozac in the runoff from chicken farms.

Our waterways won't be able to withstand this sort of abuse much longer. According to the EPA, chemical and animal waste runoff from factory farms is already responsible for more than 173,000 miles of polluted rivers and streams. The agency goes on to say, "The growing scale and concentration of [factory farms] has contributed to negative environmental and human health impacts. Pollution associated with [factory farms] degrades the quality of waters, threatens drinking water sources, and may harm air quality."

Why is liquid waste threatening our air quality? Because to get around the laws designed to protect waterways, some famers are now taking the liquid poop out of the lagoons and spraying it into the *air* instead. That's right, as we speak somewhere in this country a worker on a factory farm is taking hog poop and urine or chicken poop and pee and actually spraying it into the air. The same air that the people who live around that farm—or wherever the wind might carry it—have to breathe. A study by the Consumers Union in Texas found that the state produced over fourteen million pounds of particle dust every year that were contaminated with bacteria, fungi, and mold from animal feed and feces. And a study by the California State Senate found that animal waste lagoons "emit toxic airborne chemicals that can cause inflammatory, immune, irritation, and neurochemical problems in humans."

It's an absolutely disgusting—and dangerous—practice. Yet there aren't many other ways to deal with the massive amounts of waste produced by the animals we eat.

Every time you pick up a hamburger or order a chicken nugget, you have to realize that meat was not created in a factory or a lab. It came from a living animal, one that put a lot of stress on the environment in the short time it was alive. Maybe it was a cow emitting tons of methane into the atmosphere before it died. A pig whose feed required thousands of gallons of water to grow. A chicken whose shit was sprayed into the air, making a young child sick. No matter what kind of meat you eat, it managed to inflict plenty of damage on the environment before it made its way to your supermarket or restaurant.

YOU CAN'T EAT ANIMALS AND BE AN ENVIRONMENTALIST

> *"The food that people eat is just as important as what kind of cars they drive when it comes to creating the greenhouse-gas emissions."* —UNIVERSITY OF CHICAGO STUDY

Environmentalist wasn't a term I heard too often growing up. I remember people talking about Love Canal (a neighborhood in upstate

New York that was built on top of a chemical dump) and I watched Jacques Cousteau on TV trying to keep the oceans clean, but that was about it.

Today, awareness about the environment has risen dramatically. Organizations like Greenpeace, PETA, and Earth Justice have become very public champions for the planet. From a very early age, our children are taught the value in protecting the environment. And even though there are some crackpot politicians who like to pretend that global warming isn't real (funny how a lot of them happen to live in coal mining states, huh?), at the very least it is an issue that the vast majority of Americans are aware of.

It's inspiring to see that people are much more conscious of being sustainable than they were when I was growing up. It's not surprising that a Gallup poll found that 59 percent of Americans are either sympathetic to the environmental movement or consider themselves active environmentalists.

Odds are then that you are one of those people trying to do your part. And I salute your effort. But please consider what John Robbins has to say about the connection between eating animal products and protecting the environment:

> *Everywhere you look today, particularly in the western United States, people are seeking to conserve water. . . . These measures are prudent and helpful, but all of them combined don't save anywhere near the amount of water you would save by shifting toward a plant-based diet.*

In the documentary *Cowspiracy*, Howard Lyman, a former cattle rancher turned vegan, makes the case for giving up meat for the environment even more bluntly. "You can't be an environmentalist and eat animal products, period," says Lyman. "Kid yourself if you want; if you want to feed your addiction, so be it. But don't call yourself an environmentalist."

Many of the reasons I'll give for going vegan in this book boil down to personal choices. I can advise you to pick a diet that helps you lose weight, feel better, and reduce your chances of dying from heart disease or cancer, but ultimately it's your health.

Similarly, in the next chapter I'm going to argue that by participating in the slaughter and torture of over ten billion farm animals, you're contributing to one of the worst karmic disasters of all time. But ultimately, it's still *your* karma.

When it comes to the environment, however, it's a different story. The choices you make in this space don't affect only you. They affect your children. And your children's unborn children. Just as they're affecting me. And my children.

So please, every time you make a little step toward helping the environment, like not washing your car, consider making a much greater leap *too*. Consider all the gasses in our atmosphere, all the shit leaking into our rivers, and all the precious water being wasted that result in you eating a piece of meat, and then decide to be the hero that makes a better choice.

ALL LIVING THINGS:
DO IT FOR THE ANIMALS

"We are ingesting nightmares for breakfast, lunch, and dinner." —JOHN ROBBINS

When I was working on my book *Do You!* back in 2005, several people advised me not to include a section about the abuse of the animals. "It's going to sound preachy," they warned. "People hate hearing the 'animal rights' rap from a celebrity."

Despite their misgivings, I spoke on the issue. How could I write a book about enlightenment and not address the tens of billions of animals birthed into suffering every year? I believe that few things slow down your evolution as much as eating the meat of another being every day. It's nothing short of the biggest karmic disaster in the history of the world!

Some ten years later, there's been a shift in consciousness. Now instead of being warned to sidestep the subject, I've been asked to write an entire book about it.

I credit that shift to the passion and dedication of individuals like my guru Sharon Gannon of Jivamukti yoga. One of the translations of *guru* in the yogic tradition is "remover of darkness," and that's an accurate description of the effect Sharon had on me and countless others. I was living in the dark about what happened to the animals I was eating, and Sharon helped me see that until I confronted the truth, I was never going to get too far on the path to enlightenment.

Sharon taught me that eating animals directly contradicts one of the most basic principles, or *yamas*, of yoga, which is *ahimsa*, or "non-harming." It not only refers to avoiding physical violence between human beings but calls for compassion toward animals as well.

Practicing ahimsa is critical to our evolution because as long as we are causing harm through our actions, we're never going to achieve true happiness. "The yogi strives to cause the least amount of harm possible, and it is clear that eating a vegetarian diet causes the least harm to the planet and all creatures," she would say. "If you want to bring more peace and happiness into your own life, the method is to stop causing pain and unhappiness in the lives of others."

It's a question that should be at the front—not the back—of your mind every time you walk into the grocery store or sit down at a restaurant. Before you decide what you're going to buy or order, ask yourself this question: Am I going to make a selfish choice that causes pain? Or am I going to make a compassionate choice?

As a society, we make the selfish choice time after time. The great irony is, of course, that the unselfish choice is actually the one that's in our collective best interest.

The unselfish, compassionate choice leads directly to stronger health. The unselfish choice leads to stronger focus and energy. The unselfish choice leads to a better world for ourselves and our children.

This is why when you start studying yoga, one of the first sutras you are taught is *sthira sukham asanam*, which essentially translates to, "If we want to be free and happy, then we should not cause enslavement and unhappiness in others."

I believe the reason many people have trouble making that compassionate choice is because they don't actually make the connection between eating animal products and causing harm. We've become so desensitized to the suffering of animals that we've tricked ourselves into believing they somehow must not experience the same kind of physical suffering that we do.

If that's how you feel, then consider the role pain plays in our lives. Pain is our body's way of ordering us to withdraw from a harmful situation. We feel pain so that we know to take our hand out of a fire or move it after we've cut it with a knife. At its essence, pain is our oldest survival technique.

"There are no good reasons, scientific or philosophical, for denying that animals feel pain. If we do not doubt that other humans feel pain, we should not doubt that other animals do so too. Animals can feel pain."
—Peter Singer, *Animal Liberation*

Animals, of course, display survival techniques too. A bird flies off a branch when it hears a loud noise. Cattle stampede when they sense a predator. A bear charges if it thinks it or its cubs are in danger. They do those things because they want to live. Wouldn't it follow that they would also be able to experience pain? Especially because we know that experiencing pain is fundamental to staying alive.

Also, animals' sense of smell is stronger than that of human beings. Their sense of hearing is stronger. Their sight is stronger too. From cats to bats, their sense of touch certainly seems to be more heightened too. So if anything, it would stand to reason that animals actually feel *more* pain than humans do. Certainly not less. This is why my friend Ingrid Newkirk of PETA says, "When it comes to having a central nervous system, and the ability to feel pain, hunger, and thirst, a rat is a pig is a dog is a boy."

It's also a fish. They might not be able to scream, but there's little doubt that they feel pain, given that they have highly developed nerve sensory systems. "Have you seen how fish are able to swim in a school so precisely relating to their fish fellows and never clumsily bump into one another?" asks Sharon. "That's because they have a highly developed sense of feeling in their bodies, which enables them to feel not only the movement of the water against their skin but the presence of other beings who are close. They certainly are not cold-blooded in the sense that they are dull, insensitive, and have no feelings."

Accepting that animals experience pain should become one of your greatest motivations for going vegan. You might be able to ignore the health benefits. Or discount the environmental impact of eating meat. But when you confront head-on just how badly these animals are suffering, it becomes difficult to justify eating even *one bite* of meat.

FORGET ABOUT FARMS

> *Animals killed for their meat in America:*
> *Every minute: 38,627*
> *Every hour: 2,317,596*
> *Every day: 55,622,293*

Before I detail the torture and suffering that takes place on factory farms, I want to clear up some misconceptions about the term *farm* itself.

Ask most Americans what a farm looks like and you'll probably get pretty uniform answers: Cows grazing on rolling green hills. Pigs frolicking in the mud. Chickens pecking for feed in a yard. A farmer in overalls riding a tractor.

Those are images we've had drilled into our heads since we were kids. It's what we saw in children's books. It's what we sang about in "Old MacDonald Had a Farm." It's what we watched on TV and in the movies. Most deceptively, it's what we saw on the packaging for much of the meat and dairy we bought in the supermarkets.

Take, for example, the packaging for Perdue's Oven Stuffer roaster chicken. It features a picture of a traditional-looking white farmhouse, surrounded by trees and open fields, with a small chicken shed in the background. According to the website for the Murray Brand, the advertising firm that came up with the packaging, the image is an "iconic representation of Perdue's original family farmhouse."

You can see why they picked the picture of an old farmhouse—it's a comforting, reassuring image—but it's also a total *misrepresentation* of where that chicken came from.

Far from an idyllic family farm, most Perdue chickens are now raised in large, dimly lit, filthy-smelling sheds that hold up to thirty thousand birds. In fact, Perdue agreed to stop labeling some of its products "humanely raised" after it was sued by the Humane Society for trying to mislead customers. Perdue, argued the Humane Society, was raising chickens in conditions that "no reasonable consumer would consider 'humane.'" That's why when you pick up that Oven Stuffer roaster, you're being sold a fairy tale. A hearty side serving of propaganda to go with your poultry.

I used Perdue as an example because it's such a recognizable brand. But many other meat and dairy packagers employ a similar strategy. They show you the farm you'd like to *believe* your food came from so that you don't spend any time thinking about where it was *actually* raised. Picturing a scene like that might ruin your appetite.

To be fair, there was a time when most of the meat and dairy in this country did come from a place that looked like the Perdue farmhouse or Old MacDonald's farm of the song. Just over a hundred years ago, 99 percent of farms in this country were run by families. Cows did graze in grass fields flanked by barns. Chickens did roam free in yards. Pigs did wallow in the mud.

Those days are long, long gone. One hundred years ago, over half the workforce in the United States was employed on small, family-operated farms. Today, 99 percent of the "farms" in this country are corporate-controlled factory farms, whereas only 1 percent are still run by families. The very idea of a famer is almost obsolete. "The United

States now has more prison inmates than full-time farmers," writes Eric Schlosser in *Fast Food Nation*.

Things have changed so radically that even the government won't use the term *farm* to describe the facilities where most meat and dairy come from. Instead, the government has labeled them concentrated animal feeding operations (CAFOs). It's a term that really captures the heartlessness and industrialization of these facilities. So even though I've been using the term *factory farm*, from this point forward I'm going to follow our government's lead and switch over to CAFO. Because even just using the word *farm* to describe these hellholes lends them more dignity than they deserve.

After you've read this section, try a little experiment. Go to Google Images and do a search for "farms." The results probably look like the type of farms you like to believe meat and dairy come from. That's the fantasy you've been sold. Next, do a search for "CAFO." What you'll find is the reality. And that reality is not pretty.

As their name implies, CAFOs are built on an industrial model, where the goal is to squeeze as many animals into as little space as possible. If the people who built the slave ships had been asked to design a space to hold a hundred thousand chickens or seventy-five thousand pigs, a CAFO is what they would have come up with. And like the hold of a slave ship, conditions on most CAFOs are disgusting, inhumane, and deadly.

Sadly, the conditions I'm about to describe in detail are not isolated to a few bad apples. No matter what kind of meat you eat, a CAFO is most likely where it came from. According to Jonathan Safran Foer's *Eating Animals*, 99.9 percent of the chickens raised for meat, 99 percent of laying hens, 95 percent of pigs, and 99 percent of the turkeys on the market are from CAFOs.

This is why, the meat and dairy companies are determined to keep you from seeing—or even thinking about—what goes on inside CAFOs. They're so desperate to keep that information hidden that they've helped sponsor a series of what are known as "Ag Gag" bills. Passed in several states with the help of lobbyists, these laws make it illegal to film inside CAFOs or to even take a job at one unless you've disclosed if you've worked as an animal rights activist or journalist.

How insane is that? Employing the same level of scrutiny and paranoia you might expect from a nuclear facility, but just to work in a shed raising pigs? What could they possibly be so anxious to hide?

Well, let me tell you.

CHICKENS

> *"More than 99 percent of all chickens sold for meat in America die like this."* —JONATHAN SAFRAN FOER

Let's start with chickens, because they are the animals we eat the most of in this country. Chicken nuggets. Chicken Parmesan. Fried chicken. Chicken fingers. Jerked chicken. General Tso's chicken. Chicken soup with rice. Chicken and waffles. I could go on and on.

According to the National Chicken Council, the average American eats over eighty-six pounds of the bird every year. Collectively, we eat over seven billion chickens every year. Americans ate *1.25 billion* chicken wings during the 2015 Super Bowl alone. Enough chicken wings to stretch from Seattle to Boston and back again—twenty-eight times over.

But where do all those birds come from? And how are they raised?

Almost all chickens are born inside incubators in huge hatcheries. A few days after birth they're packed into crates and shipped out to CAFOs. "OK, what's the big deal about that?" you might say. The big deal is that being separated from their mothers is very traumatic for chicks. After all, what do we often call a human who is particularly nurturing? That's right, a *mother hen*. We get that term from real hens, who are incredibly engaged with their offspring. There's no doubt that forced separation is an incredibly distressing experience for both hen and chick.

Once they're shipped out, chicks are divided into two groupings: broilers (which provide most of the chicken meat we eat) and eggs hens, which produce the eggs.

Let's check out the life of a typical broiler first.

Broilers

> *"Broilers now grow so rapidly that the heart and lungs are not developed well enough to support the remainder of the body, resulting in congestive heart failure and tremendous death losses."* —FEEDSTUFFS, AGRICULTURAL TRADE NEWSPAPER

After arriving at a CAFO, broilers are crammed into huge sheds—or "grower houses"—that house tens of thousands of other birds. Right off the bat, this makes the chicks disoriented because in nature they're raised in small groups of fewer than a hundred. Again, that might not seem like a big deal, but what do we call a very structured social hierarchy? That's right, a *pecking order*. Another term we've borrowed from the chicken world. (For a bunch of birds that are often written off as "stupid," humans sure seem to get a lot of social inspiration from them, huh?)

Having their natural pecking order destroyed is so stressful for the birds that they often begin to attack each other or even themselves with their beaks. Because of this tendency, when the birds are just a couple days old they have half their beaks seared off in a process known in the industry as "debeaking." Or as I call it, cutting off part of a chick's face without any painkillers.

Conditions inside the grower houses are absolutely hellish. Imagine fifty thousand chickens inside a massive enclosed warehouse-like shed, without any windows to let in fresh air or sunlight. The air is thick with the smell of chicken shit (which eventually turns into ammonia). The only circulation comes from huge fans in the walls. The space is kept dark most of the day in order to save money and to slow down the rate at which the males reach sexual maturity.

This is how Michael Specter, a writer for the *New Yorker*, described walking into one such grower house:

> I was almost knocked to the ground by the overpowering smell of ammonia and feces. My eyes burned and so did my lungs, and I could neither see nor breathe. . . . There must have been 30,000 chickens sitting on the floor silently in front of me. They didn't move, they didn't cluck. They were almost like statues of chickens,

living in near total darkness. And they would spend every minute of their six-week lives that way.

Because of these unnatural and unhealthy conditions, many chicks become sick and die slow, agonizing deaths. Some catch infections after their beaks are chopped off. Others literally can't walk to water stations because their legs don't work (a common condition because of inbreeding). Others get sick from the various diseases that result from packing so many animals into so little space. Still more go crazy from being confined in darkness and eventually die from stress.

Despite all these aliments, the birds don't receive any medical help. If a chicken gets sick from infection and falls to the floor, covered in shit and gasping for breath, there isn't a veterinarian who tries to treat it. Instead, that chicken dies a slow death where it lies. When it finally passes, its carcass is just left to rot.

For the first few weeks of their lives, the birds that survive the shock and danger of being born into such an environment have a little bit of space to move around in. As they collectively grow, however, that space begins to rapidly disappear. Often by the time they're just a few weeks old, they're packed in so tightly that they literally don't have room to flap their wings. Not that they could fly anywhere even if they could. From the time they arrive at the hatchery to when they're taken to slaughter, these birds never go outside or even see the natural light of day.

The chickens grow much bigger—and faster—than they ever did in the past. In 1923, it took 112 days to raise a chicken to reach a slaughter weight of about five pounds. Today, broilers reach the same weight after just 47 days. To help understand just how unnatural a growth spurt that is, a report by the University of Arkansas says the human equivalent would be a human weighing 350 pounds by the time he or she turned two years old.

Why are we forcing these birds to grow so big so fast? The same reason we feed them antibiotics: Americans prefer fattier meat. To achieve that, growers give birds feed that is laced with hormones, antibiotics, and other chemicals that speed up their growth rate.

The result is what you could call Frankenstein's monster chickens, birds that were designed and altered by scientists, not by nature. Most broilers' breasts become so oversize that by the time they're several weeks old they'll topple over if they try to walk. Craig Watts, longtime Perdue supplier who called out the company for misrepresenting the conditions its chickens are raised in, describes to Al Jazeera his birds' inability to walk: "It's three steps and flop. . . . That's what they're bred to do." Most spend their remaining days sitting in their own feces on the floor of a darkened grow house.

The end result might be a tastier chicken breast, but remember the cost required to achieve it. Be awake the next time you go into the poultry aisle at your supermarket. Make a point of noticing how all the chicken wings, or whole birds, are almost identical in size and weight. That should tip you off that something isn't right.

Look at your family. Or your neighbors. Or your coworkers. Is everyone the same height and weight? Does everyone have the same size breasts? Or thighs? Or legs? Of course not. Some people are big, some are scrawny. When you look on the chicken shelf, every single bird is like a LeBron James or a Serena Williams—a "perfect" physical specimen. That sort of uniformity can happen only through manipulation and drugs.

If there's any good news here, it's that broilers don't have to live in their awful conditions for long. Despite enjoying a life span of up to fifteen to twenty years in the wild, most broilers are ready to be slaughtered after just six weeks.

It's not surprising that the slaughter process is just as horrific as the conditions in which the birds were raised. In his meticulously researched book *Eating Animals*, Foer details the process. The journey to death starts with the birds being pulled from the grow houses by their legs and stuffed into crates, often leaving them with broken bones. Those crates are then loaded onto trucks and taken to a slaughterhouse, a trip that often takes hours. Since the birds are on their way to be killed, they aren't given food or water or protected from the elements. It's such a brutal trip many of them die before they even make it to the slaughterhouse.

Once they finally arrive, the birds are dumped from their crates onto long conveyor belts, where workers grab them and then hang them upside down by their legs in shackles. By this point the chickens, as you can imagine, are freaking out. They try—unsuccessfully—to break free from their chains, which only leads to more broken bones. The petrified birds also defecate on themselves. As they struggle, they're dragged through a pool of electrified water, intended to knock them unconscious before they're killed.

After the bath, the birds are then dragged across a rotating blade that is meant to slit their throat. If the bird is "lucky," it will already be unconscious and will experience a clean cut that will cause it to bleed to death in a matter of minutes.

Sadly, many birds aren't so lucky. Because they weren't fully knocked out by their dip in the pool, they're still thrashing as they pass over the blade. This often leads to "improper" cuts that leave the birds injured but alive. It happens often enough that slaughterhouses employ "kill men" whose job it is to manually slit the throats of the birds that haven't been killed properly by the automated blade. But in plants where 175 birds are killed every minute, it's often impossible for the kill men to keep up.

That's terrible, because the next stop for the birds is a tank of scalding water, designed to boil off their feathers. But Charles Painter, a federal poultry inspector, tells the *Washington Post* that many chickens aren't dead when they reach that hellish broth. "They are literally throwing the birds into the shackles, often breaking their legs as they do it. They are working so fast they sometimes get just one leg in the shackles. When that happens, the chickens aren't hanging right. . . . They don't get killed, and they go into the scald tank alive."

According to the National Chicken Council, an industry group, roughly 180 million chickens are killed "improperly" every year. Since that number comes from an industry that polices itself (chickens aren't protected under the Humane Methods of Livestock Slaughter Act) one can only imagine what the real number is.

After they're taken out of the water, the birds' feet and heads are removed and their guts are pulled out. Removing the guts has to be done carefully, otherwise feces will contaminate the rest of the carcass. But since workers are cutting open hundreds of birds an hour, mistakes are often made.

In the past, inspectors had to reject any carcasses they saw contaminated by feces. Recently, however, the chicken industry got the USDA to reclassify fecal smears as "cosmetic blemishes" and inspectors are now allowed to let those birds pass. Think about that the next time you bite into some chicken breast.

The inspectors work under conditions that almost ensure unsanitary birds get shipped to the public. On average, inspectors have all of two seconds to look at a bird as it goes past them on an assembly line. Two seconds to check each of twenty-five thousand birds a day for deformities, fecal smears, puss stains, and cancer tumors. So you can imagine how thorough those "checks" are.

Scott Bronstein, a reporter for the *Atlanta Journal Constitution*, interviewed hundreds of USDA inspectors about working in a slaughterhouse and afterward reported, "Every week millions of chickens leaking yellow pus, stained by green feces, contaminated by harmful bacteria, or marred by lung and heart infections, cancerous tumors, or skin conditions are shipped for sale to consumers." But hey, what's the Super Bowl without chicken wings, right?

As nasty as all that sounds, there's still one more part of this revolting process. Before the chicken carcasses can be shipped out, they have to be chilled. The easiest way to do that would be to refrigerate them, but cold air causes their bodies to lose weight, which would decrease their value.

So instead of chilling the carcasses, they're dumped in a vat of cold water, which is absorbed into their bodies. That makes the meat heavier—and more profitable. The problem is that when one dirty bird covered in bacteria and feces is dumped into the water, it pollutes the water for all the birds that come after it. This happens so often that those water tanks are often called "fecal soup" in the industry.

After being dumped in the contaminated soup, the carcass has to be submerged in a chlorine bath in order to kill the germs it's been exposed to. Even still, Foer reports that between 35 and 75 percent of chickens sold in stores still contain some level of the *E. coli* bacteria.

> "In our latest analysis of fresh, whole broilers bought at stores nationwide, two-thirds harbored salmonella and/or campylobacter, the leading bacterial causes of food-borne disease."
> —*Consumer Reports*, 2010

It might seem like I'm trying to gross you out with this information, but I'm simply informing you about a process you're already a party to. That chicken nugget arrives on your plate cut up into cute little shapes to distract you from even thinking about where that meat came from. From all the inhumane and unnatural things that happened to it before it reached your plate.

Again, the conditions I just described don't represent a few bad apples or the exceptions to the rule. If you ate a chicken nugget or chicken wing or piece of fried chicken recently, it is almost certain that bird was subjected to this suffering.

Layer Hens

> *"Without a doubt,* laying hens *are the most* abused *animals in all of farming."*
>
> —MASSACHUSETTS SOCIETY FOR THE PREVENTION
> OF CRUELTY TO ANIMALS

I wish I was done with chickens, but that was just broilers. What happens to the chickens that lay your eggs is just as bad. If not worse.

Though you may not be aware of it, "layer" chickens are actually a different breed from broilers and are raised exclusively for their eggs. At any given time there are *three hundred million* layers in captivity, providing the eggs for everything from your omelets to French toast to huevos rancheros to custard pie.

Once layer chicks arrive at a CAFO, they're put on a conveyor belt and separated by sex. For male chicks, they've already reached the end of the line. Unable to produce eggs, they hold no value and are immediately "disposed" of; the "lucky" ones are thrown into huge grinding machines that chop them up in a few seconds. The unlucky ones are killed manually, which investigations have revealed often means being clubbed to death, or stomped on by workers. Sometimes the male chicks are simply thrown in trash cans and left to slowly die of starvation.

For the females, the suffering has just begun. Once at the CAFO, they're crammed into wire "battery cages," where they'll spend the rest of their lives with ten other hens, each in a space no bigger than an eight-by-eleven-inch piece of paper. (For a sense of how confining that is, a grown hen's wingspan is thirty-six inches.) Since living in such tight conditions often drives the hens to violence and even cannibalism, their beaks are also clipped off. Again, without any painkillers.

The cages the hens live in are stacked on top of each other, often several rows high. That means the hens on the bottom levels spend their entire lives literally being pissed and shat on by the birds above them.

When the hens are around twenty-six weeks old, they're artificially inseminated so that they can begin laying eggs. After being inseminated, they're kept in complete darkness for several weeks. Then the lights inside their sheds are turned on for up to twenty hours a day. The combined effect is to make the birds think it's spring, which is when they naturally lay eggs. By manipulating the lighting this way, the factories can get the chickens to do the unnatural and lay eggs year-round. CAFO chickens lay around three hundred eggs a year, almost three times as many as they would otherwise.

In the wild, hens also go out of their way to find a private, safe place to lay their eggs. But that's impossible when they're confined to a cage surrounded by thousands of other birds. "The worst torture to which a battery hen is exposed is the inability to retire somewhere for the laying act," the Nobel Prize–winning scientist Dr. Konrad Lorenz told the Humane Society. "For the person who knows something about animals it is truly heart-rending to watch how a chicken tries again and again to crawl beneath her fellow cage mates to search there in vain for cover."

"When people ask me why I don't eat meat or any other animal products, I say, 'Because they are unhealthy and they are the product of a violent and inhumane industry.'"
—Casey Affleck, actor

For two years the hens are kept in a vicious circle of being insemi-nated and laying eggs. Once they're unable to produce any more eggs, their value to the manufacturer is gone. That's when the birds are sent off to the slaughterhouse, to be transported and killed in the same brutal manner as the broilers.

The layer hens are so beat up that by the time they're slaughtered, the CAFOs won't even sell their meat for general consumption. In-stead, the flesh is deemed fit only for chicken noodle soup, animal food, or the National School Lunch Program. Think about that next time your kid tells you they were served chicken salad or chicken tacos in the school cafeteria.

Before I move on, a quick word about "free-range" and "cage-free" chickens. It's become popular to believe that by buying only free-range or cage-free products you've somehow removed yourself from the ter-rible suffering a typical broiler or layer undergoes.

Sorry, but as with almost everything else in the food industries, "free-range" and "cage-free" are just marketing devices that don't re-flect reality. It would be great if *free-range* meant the chicken you bought spent its life ranging freely on a farm somewhere. But of course it didn't. To label eggs free-range, all a company has to do is provide its chickens with "access to the outdoors." That's it.

Most companies follow the letter of that law but not the spirit. That means if a grower has a hangar with twenty-five thousand chickens in it, as long as there is a little door at one end of it leading to the outdoors, it's OK to label those birds free-range. As Foer points out, it wouldn't matter if that door led to only a patch of dirt no bigger than your bedroom. As long as the chickens technically have access to it, they're free-range. "The free-range label is *bullshit*," he declares in *Eating Animals*. "It should provide no more peace of mind than 'all-natural,' 'fresh,' or 'magical.'"

Cage-free isn't much better. Yes, it is an improvement that those hens aren't kept stacked in cages. But just because they're not in cages doesn't mean they've "flown the coop." Instead, they're still kept packed into sheds with tens of thousands of other birds, still forced to fight for a piece of living space not much bigger than a piece of paper. They just don't have to live with a steady stream of piss and shit raining down on them all day. They're still all debeaked when they're young, drugged throughout their lives, and ultimately slaughtered just like "regular" birds.

Unless you have a chicken coop in your backyard, every time you eat eggs, cage-free or not, you're still contributing to this cycle of suffering.

COWS

Like layer hens and broiler chickens, cows are divided into two main groups: milk and beef. And just as with chickens, both types suffer greatly for our appetites. Let's start with dairy cows.

Dairy Cows

> *"Far from leading the carefree lives portrayed in the dairy industry's 'happy cow' commercials, the vast majority of cows used for dairy production today lead lives of deprivation, confinement, painful mutilations, and cruel handling."* —MERCY FOR ANIMALS

Shortly after birth, the calves are separated from their mothers, which is incredibly traumatic. Many calves stop eating out of fear and cry for their mothers so hard and for so long their throats become raw. I have a friend who spent some time on a cattle farm and he said the sound of a calf crying for its mother throughout the night is one of the most heartbreaking things he'd ever heard. He described it as pure emotion, like someone mourning at the funeral of a family member who was gone too soon.

Since they can't produce milk, male calves have little value to dairy CAFOs (I almost wrote *farmers* but caught myself). As a result, many are raised as veal, the term for male calves whose flesh is kept tender by denying them solid foods or exercise. For the entirety of their short lives, veal calves are kept tied down in small pens barely bigger than their bodies. They're restrained to prevent them from making any movements that could help them build up muscles. They're kept on a liquid diet intended to keep their flesh soft, but often leaves them near death from chronic diarrhea. After almost four months of living this nightmare, off to the slaughterhouse they go.

We put veal through all of that suffering and trauma just to "enjoy" a soft piece of meat. Wow. I've always said you have to be a little sick in the head to eat veal. But truth be told it's not like life is that significantly better for the female calves raised for their milk.

After being forcibly separated from their mothers, the female calves are isolated in tiny pens for several weeks before being moved to a larger pen with other calves. Even there, each calf has only thirty-five square feet of room to move about. Remember, calves weigh almost a hundred pounds at birth. So that's asking an animal larger than most adolescents to spend its entire day in a space that's probably smaller than your bathroom.

The calves are also subjected to a process called "dehorning," in which workers attempt to remove horn tissue from the animals' heads to prevent them from growing actual horns when they're older. The techniques used are barbaric. Workers dig tissue out with a sharp instrument, burn it out with chemicals, or cut tissue that's started to grow with shears. All the methods are incredibly painful. According to a report by NBC news, only 10 percent of cows get any sort of painkiller or receive medical treatment after being dehorned.

For food, the cows are fed feed laced with antibiotics and growth hormones. In addition to keeping the cows from getting sick in such squalid conditions, the antibiotics also increase milk production, as do the hormones. This drug cocktail makes the cows susceptible to a host of illnesses, including lameness.

Once they're old enough to breed, the cows are moved into individual stalls. These stalls, basically fenced-in concrete slabs not much bigger than a cow's body, will be their homes for the rest of their lives.

With no room to move or even turn around, the cows are forced to stand in their own waste day after day, over time rotting their hooves black. Despite whatever image may be on your milk carton or your container of half-and-half, there's no grazing on green hills for most dairy cows. Few ever see natural sunlight again, let alone grass.

There also aren't any farmers sitting on overturned buckets, patiently milking cows by hand. Nope, that's not how we get milk anymore. Instead, several times a day the cows are hooked up to a machine that pumps the milk from their udders. The stress caused by these machines often leads to mastitis, a very painful condition that causes the cow's udders to swell and leak puss. According to PETA, up to 50 percent of dairy cows suffer from it. Women sometimes get mastitis after giving birth—any of you who have experienced it know just how painful it can be. Especially if it's left untreated, as it often is with dairy cows. Many of their udders become so swollen and distended that it looks like they have a giant balloon stuck to their stomachs, making it almost impossible for the cows to stand or walk.

Because a dairy cow's only value to a CAFO lies in its ability to produce milk, they are kept in an almost nonstop cycle of pregnancy, birth, and milking. Like humans, a cow's pregnancy lasts roughly nine months. But because cows can conceive again during their "nursing" period, the average dairy cow is artificially impregnated twice within a twelve-month period. This aggressive approach—combined with the increased milk flow that comes from antibiotics and growth hormones—allows dairy cows to produce almost twenty-two thousand pounds of milk each year, almost double what they produced forty years ago.

Ladies, imagine being forced to be pregnant twice every twelve months, year after year after year. While eating an unhealthy diet laced with drugs. Your body would just give out after a while, right? Well, that's exactly what happens to most dairy cows.

Even though a cow's natural life span is up to twenty years, the cycle of pregnancy and milking that the cows are subjected to is so exhausting that most are considered spent by the time they're just five years old. So off to the slaughterhouse they go as well, where their worn-out bodies are turned into hamburger meat.

Beef Cows

> "I've seen guys punch cows, stick cattle prods in their eyes, bragging, 'I got her in the eyeball!'"
>
> —UNDERCOVER ANIMAL ACTIVIST TO *ROLLING STONE*

Like dairy cows, calves raised for their beef are separated from their mothers shortly after birth. If that weren't traumatic enough, they're then forced to undergo several torturous procedures. First they're marked with a red-hot branding iron. Then, because it's thought to increase meat tenderness, the males are castrated. In some cases their testicles are sliced off with a blade. In others their testicles are tied off with string and denied blood until they simply fall off. Both the branding and castrations are performed without painkillers.

You can tell yourself that castration must not be too painful, but any man reading this knows that can't be true. I could offer a million dollars to the first man out there who would let their testicles be cut off—or tied off—without painkillers and probably not one of you would take me up on it. So don't tell me those calves aren't being tortured something awful.

For their first several months the calves live in facilities called "range lands" where they are afforded space to move around. At around one year old they're trucked to feedlots, where they are fattened up until they're ready to be slaughtered.

The cows are usually around six hundred pounds when they arrive at a feedlot, but need to get up to twelve hundred pounds, or market weight, in the next several months. To achieve this rapid increase, their diet is switched from grass to grain. The grain, which they're fed three times a day, is laced with antibiotics and hormones to speed up their growth even quicker. Since cows were never designed to eat grain, this diet makes them very sick. Most live cows live with chronic digestive pain—sort of like having a stomachache that never goes away. The *Journal of Animal Science* reports that this grain-based diet also creates liver abscesses in up to 32 percent of beef cattle, a condition that is often fatal.

Feedlots are massive facilities that often stretch farther than the eye can see, some containing over a hundred thousand cows. Because the cows are no longer eating grass, they're packed into dirt-floored holding pens, where they spend their days standing in their own shit. They aren't offered any protection from the elements, which results in many cows on feedlots in southern states dying from heatstroke, while many farther north die from exposure during the winter.

After roughly two hundred days on the feedlot, the cows are ready for slaughter. Even though feedlots are scattered around the country, the actual slaughtering is done at only a handful of facilities. This means that cows often have to travel between twelve and fifteen hundred miles to reach their death. As with chickens, it's a brutal journey. By law, the trucks, in which the cows are packed in like slaves, can travel for twenty-eight straight hours without stopping for rest. This means cows often go the entire trip without receiving any food, water, or medical care.

The cows arrive at the slaughterhouse exhausted and terrified. Many of them can no longer walk because they were sick before the journey started. Animals in this condition are known as "downer cows" and by federal law, cannot be killed for food. Despite this, slaughterhouses go to great lengths to encourage the downers to move again. Some have chains tied around their legs and are dragged from the trucks. Others are poked with electrical rods—sometimes in their anus—to try to make them stand. There are reports of workers—apparently inspired by the torture techniques employed at Abu Gharib—sticking water hoses down the downers' throats to make them stand. Some facilities will even pick up downers with forklifts to try to get them back on their feet.

Even though the fact that the government has deemed downers unfit for human consumption (they are three times more likely to have *E. coli*), cows in this condition are slaughtered all of the time. In 2007, an investigation conducted by the Humane Society found that the Westland/Hallmark Meat Packing Company in Southern California had processed thirty-seven million pounds of downer beef. And who did they sell all that "unfit" beef to? The Department of Agriculture, which in turn sent it to the National School Lunch Program. How disgusting is that?

Once the cows—downers and more healthy ones—are forced out of the trucks, they're herded into a single-file line and led into the actual slaughterhouse. Inside, they're forced onto a conveyor belt, where metal gates close in from the sides in an effort to keep them from moving around too much.

After a short trip, they walk up a ramp (sadistically referred to as the "Stairway to Heaven" in some slaughterhouses) and are met by a worker operating a bolt gun, which uses compressed air to fire a metal bolt. As the belt slows to a stop, the worker fires the bolt into the cow's skull from point-blank range. The bolt won't puncture the skull, but will—in theory—render the cow unconscious for what's going to happen to it next.

Unfortunately, as we've learned, things don't always go as planned in slaughterhouses. Maybe the cow, sensing something is about to happen, flinches at the last second and the bolt misses. Maybe the gun misfires. Or maybe the worker is distracted and hits the cow in the wrong spot. As in poultry, beef slaughterhouses process a huge amount of cows, sometimes up to four hundred an hour. The worker with the bolt gun is never going to have the luxury to take his or her time and make sure that every cow is truly knocked out before it's passed on to the butcher.

The butcher's job is to sever the cow's throat and then begin to cut its body apart. Unfortunately, many cows are still conscious while this is happening. A longtime slaughterhouse butcher tells the *Washington Post* that he was often forced to cut the legs off of completely conscious cows rather than risk slowing down the assembly line. "They blink. They make noises," he said. "The head moves, the eyes are wide and looking around. . . . They die piece by piece."

Ritual slaughterhouses, the kind that butcher kosher meat and halal meat, have a reputation for being more humane. Unfortunately, it's not well earned. If anything, cows often suffer even worse at those facilities. A PETA investigation of kosher slaughterhouses between 2004 and 2008 found that workers at numerous plants were cutting cow's throats while the animals were fully conscious and leaving them to bleed to death slowly. In her book *Thinking in Pictures*, animal activist Dr. Temple Grandin describes a ritual slaughter she witnessed at a kosher facility:

> *Prior to slaughter, live cattle were hung upside down by a chain attached to one back leg. It was so horrible I could not stand to watch it. The frantic bellows of terrified cattle could be heard in both the office and the parking lot. Sometimes an animal's back leg was broken during hoisting.*

Even if you can't find much empathy for these "wide-eyed and terrified" animals, understand that the horror they experience before being slaughtered is potentially going to affect your health.

Cows are extremely cautious animals by nature. Changes in environment, loud noises, and rough handling all stress them out. That means during the long ride to the slaughterhouse, a cow is going to be scared out of its mind. It's going to be frightened as it's herded into the chutes. It's going to be downright terrified listening to the cows before it bellowing as they're killed. Essentially from the moment it is taken from the feedlot to the moment it is killed, a cow is pumping adrenaline, cortisol, and other fear-associated steroids into its body. Steroids that are still in the cow's meat when it's consumed by a human. I remember the rapper KRS-One speaking on this phenomenon in his 1990 song "Beef":

> See cows live under fear and stress
> Trying to think what's gonna happen next
> Fear and stress can become a part of you
> In your cells and blood, this is true
> So when the cow is killed, believe it
> You preserve those cells, you freeze it
> Thaw it out with the blood and season it
> Then you sit down and begin eatin it
> In your body, it's structure becomes your structure
> All the fear and stress of another

I didn't really get what KRS was rhyming about back then, but I damn sure get it now: People are bringing stress and fear into their own lives by eating the stress and fear of cows. Twenty-five years after KRS tried to warn us, researchers in Europe are starting to find that there does appear to be a correlation between the stress animals experience and issues with human growth, especially with the reproductive system. So remember, the cruel and barbaric way that a cow was killed isn't only a moral issue: It's also potentially affecting your health.

Eating fear isn't the only way beef is making you sick. According to the CDC, between 2009 and 2013 at least seventy-five outbreaks of *E. coli* were traced back to our beef supply. The strand of *E. coli* most commonly associated with beef is estimated to cause ninety-six thousand illnesses, thirty-two hundred hospitalizations, and thirty-one deaths in the United States each year. All that sickness and death also costs us $405 million a year in health-care expenses.

How is so much *E. coli* getting in our beef? The bacteria grows naturally in a cow's stomach, intestines, and manure (though it grows faster in cows that eat grain instead of grass). When a cow is butchered, it's critical that the stomach and intestines are removed carefully, so bacteria doesn't contaminate the rest of the carcass. But workers who are butchering hundreds of cows an hour don't have the luxury to be careful. Here's how Eric Schlosser describes what often happens:

> *The slaughterhouses that the United States have are pretty unique in terms of the speed of production. We have slaughterhouses that will process 300, 400 cattle an hour, which is as much as twice as many as anywhere else in the world. And it's that speed of production that can lead to food-safety problems. When workers are working very quickly, they may make mistakes. It's during the evisceration of the animal, or the removal of the hide, that manure can get on the meat. And when manure gets on some meat, and then that meat is ground up with lots of other meat, the whole lot of it can be contaminated.*

It's a process that doesn't only leave consumers vulnerable to *E. coli* but also endangers workers at the slaughterhouses. The Human Rights Watch has reported that slaughterhouse workers have the most dangerous job in America. "The meatpacking industry not only has the highest injury rate, but also has by far the highest rate of serious injury," says Schlosser. "Five more than five times the national average, as measured in lost workdays."

Dangerous conditions aren't just limited to beef slaughterhouses. A study by the Southern Poverty Law Center (SPLC) found that 72 percent of poultry workers it surveyed had suffered a serious injury on the job. Workers using blades accidently cut off their own fingers or suffer deep wounds. Those with repetitive tasks like deboning meat or twisting off chicken wings often report repetitive stress injuries. A worker who had to twist off eighteen thousand chicken wings a day told the SPLC that after a month on the job he'd developed carpal tunnel syndrome so severe he couldn't use his hands anymore. He was fired.

The U.S. Bureau of Labor Statistics (BLS) says the injury and illness rates for the meatpacking industry is almost two and a half times higher than the national average. Still, the number of workers injured at slaughterhouses is probably much greater than we even know. Many of the workers are immigrants from Mexico, Central America, and Somalia, who are afraid to report injuries out of fear they will be fired or deported. Because bosses know the workers likely won't complain or file reports, they are worked relentlessly and paid poorly. In the 1970s, meatpacking had one of the lowest turnover rates in the country. Today, according to Schlosser, "it has the highest turnover rate of any industrial job."

PIGS

"It's like eating my niece!"

—CAMERON DIAZ, AFTER LEARNING THAT PIGS

ARE AS SMART AS A THREE-YEAR-OLD

Some people are able to ignore the suffering of animals like chickens and cows by saying, "Those are stupid animals." It's not even remotely true, but it's a convenient attitude for people to hold on to.

No one can make that claim about pigs, though. Pigs are really smart. Without question smarter than your dog. No offense, but smarter than your two-year-old child too.

In an article celebrating their intelligence, the *New York Times* wrote, "Pigs are among the quickest of animals to learn a new routine, and pigs can do a circus's worth of tricks: jump hoops, bow and stand, spin and make wordlike sounds on command, roll out rugs, herd sheep, close and open cages, play videogames with joysticks, and more."

Pigs might be smarter than most domesticated animals, but they aren't treated any better. The conditions pigs are kept in on CAFOs, some of which hold more than ten thousand animals, are incredibly inhumane. This is how *Rolling Stone* writer Jeff Tietz describes a CAFO run by Smithfield Foods, one of the largest pork producers in the country:

> *Forty fully grown 250-pound male hogs often occupy a pen the size of a tiny apartment. They trample each other to death. There is no sunlight, straw, fresh air, or earth. The floors are slatted to allow excrement to fall into a catchment pit under the pens, but many things besides excrement can wind up in the pits: afterbirths, piglets accidently crushed by their mothers, old batteries, broken bottles of insecticide, antibiotic syringes, stillborn pigs—anything small enough to fit through the foot-wide pipes that drain the pits. . . .*
>
> *The temperature inside hog houses is often hotter than ninety degrees. The air, saturated almost to the point of precipitation with gases from shit and chemicals, can be lethal to the pigs. Enormous exhaust fans run twenty-four hours a day. The ventilation systems*

function like the ventilators of terminal patients: If they break
down for any length of time, pigs start dying.

As bad as that sounds, those pens still sound like luxury condos compared to the conditions female pigs, or sows, are forced to live in. Once
sows are old enough to breed, some are artificially inseminated. Others
are confined to what is known in the industry as "rape racks": tiny
stalls where male pigs are given access to sows who have no space to
move away or escape.

After being inseminated, pregnant sows are put in a "gestation
crate." These are essentially a metal cage seven feet by two feet. They're
so narrow that the sow is never even able to turn around, let alone
walk. Except for when she gives birth, this crate will be the sow's home
for the next several years, until it's time to be slaughtered. Dr. Temple
Grandin compares the experience of being forced to live in a gestation
crate to spending your entire life stuck in an airline seat (an economy
one at that).

This is how Matthew Scully, a former speechwriter for President
George W. Bush (hardly the type of guy you'd expect to criticize the meat
industry), describes one of the cages in an article for the *National Review*:

> *Living creatures, every bit as intelligent and sensitive as dogs, lie*
> *trapped by the millions in a sunless hell of metal and concrete, for*
> *years unable to walk or turn around, afforded not even straw to*
> *lie on—because even that little kindness, like giving the pigs extra*
> *space, would throw off the miserly economics of the enterprise. All*
> *of this, we are emphatically assured, is right and necessary—not*

only for the sake of more cost-efficient production, holding down the all-important price of bacon, but also for the benefit of the animals themselves. Does anybody really believe this, even the people who insist that it is true?

Thankfully, several states have already banned the use of gestation crates, and some major pork buyers like Wendy's and McDonald's have said they'll stop buying from producers that use them (though McDonald's won't totally phase them out till 2022). Companies who still use gestation crates are trying to avoid criticism by rebranding them as "individual maternity pens." They can call them whatever they want, but they're still torture chambers that should be outlawed.

Speaking of torture, shortly after piglets are born, they have their teeth snipped off with pliers. This is done to prevent injury later when the pigs inevitably start fighting in their cramped quarters. For the same reason, they also have their tails cut off. Snipping the pig's teeth and cutting off their tails are both performed without painkillers.

For male piglets, there's an additional torture to endure: that's right, castration. Because adolescent pigs develop a scent many meat eaters find unappetizing, male piglets have their testicles ripped off shortly after birth. And yes, this procedure is performed by hand and without painkillers. Noticing a trend here?

I wish I could report that the method used to kill pigs breaks the torturous trend we've already seen with chickens and cows, but if anything, it's worse. Like chickens and cows, pigs are jammed into trucks and driven to the slaughterhouse. The conditions in these trucks are particularly barbaric: workers have described pigs being packed in so tightly that some stomachs exploded from the pressure. Like chickens and cows, pigs on the way to slaughter are denied food and water and are left exposed to the elements.

Once they arrive at the slaughtering house—or "rendering plant" as they're called in the industry—they're herded into huge holding pens, where they're packed so tightly that some suffocate to death. After being separated into groups of three or four, they're ushered into a room where a worker with a bolt gun awaits them. On the Humane Society's website there's a video called "Iowa Pig Slaughterhouse," which depicts what comes next. In the clip, the worker walks up to each pig and fires a bolt into its head. Despite the blow, many of the pigs aren't knocked out. Instead, they writhe around in agony on the floor after being shot. Some even get back up on their feet and begin to stagger around, only to be shot again. Even after being shot a second time, they are still conscious.

That's where the video ends, but we know what happens next: The pigs, some still screaming and struggling, are hung upside down on metal racks and have their throats slit. After being left to bleed out for a couple of minutes, they are transported via a trolley system to huge vats of scalding-hot water, in which they're submerged in order to remove their skin and hair. Despite being stunned and having had their throats slit, many are still alive when this happens.

Not surprisingly, a former slaughterhouse worker tells PETA that pigs being boiled alive is an everyday occurrence. "There's no way these animals can bleed out in the few minutes it takes to get up the ramp," he says, referring to the trolley system that takes them to the tanks. "By the time they hit the scalding tank, they're still fully conscious and squealing. Happens all the time." Again, the rush for profit is a major factor: "Rendering plants" often kill upwards of 1,000 pigs an hour.

I'm sickened when I think about how any animal is killed, but I'm extra outraged by what happens to these pigs. As I said, these are highly intelligent animals.

As a culture, we love and cherish dogs because they can sit on command and fetch sticks. Some will even give you a paw. Can you imagine the esteem we'd have for them if they could play video games too? A pig can do all that and more. Yet for some reason we don't afford them even a fraction of the same love, respect, and humanity we heap upon dogs.

You probably remember when the football star Michael Vick was sentenced to twenty-three months behind bars for running a dog-fighting operation in which pit bulls he owned were brutally tortured and killed. At the time, I joined many other people in speaking out against what Vick had done and the sport of dogfighting in general.

Yet it needs to be said that if you were outraged by Vick, but still eat animal products yourself, then you are a hypocrite. Sorry if that sounds harsh, but I don't see any other way to call it.

If you were disgusted by how Vick treated those dogs, then please understand that every single piece of pork or bacon that you eat comes from an animal that was tortured and killed in a manner every bit as brutal as those dogs were.

Let's be real: If there were a *single* facility treating puppies and dogs the way we treat pigs—pulling out their teeth and castrating them without painkillers, keeping them confined to crates for years on end, cutting their throats while they're still conscious, and boiling them while they were still alive—the outrage would be deafening. There would be protests, and the people who owned the CAFOs and rendering plants would be thrown in jail. Op-ed pieces would be written in every newspaper and stringent new laws would be passed. As well they should be.

But when a hundred million pigs are tortured and killed in the ways I just described, we largely accept it. Yes, there are courageous advocates like the Humane Society, PETA, and Animal Sanctuary who speak out, but their voices are lost in the silence of our collective indifference.

Many years ago I was watching the *Texas Chainsaw Massacre* with Kimora. After we finished watching a scene where a screaming woman was fleeing the chain-saw guy, Kimora turned to me and said, "You know, this kinda makes me appreciate vegetarians." "How so?" I asked her. "Because if animals could talk, they would all be screaming like that woman before they got slaughtered. And because they can't, we just assume it's OK." My prayer for this book is that it helps you have a similar moment of clarity. A realization that just because animals can't tell us otherwise doesn't mean they don't suffer. It's time we heard the shrieks, bellows, and cries of these animals who can't speak for themselves.

FISH

> *"Even though fish don't scream [audibly to humans] when they are in pain and anguish, their behavior should be evidence enough of their suffering when they are hooked or netted. They struggle, endeavoring to escape, and, by so doing, demonstrate they have a will to survive."*
>
> —DR. MICHAEL FOX

I need to say a quick word about fish. To a lot of folks, eating fish doesn't seem as bad as eating other kinds of meat. But as I already mentioned, fish feel pain. So if you stick a piece of sharp metal through their mouth, they're going to feel that. If you pull them up out of the sea and leave them on a ship's deck to suffocate—which is how almost every commercially caught fish dies—they will suffer an incredibly painful death.

It's also important to know that when you eat a piece of fish, you're contributing to the suffering of dozens of other animals too. Why? Commercial fishing isn't done by hand. Instead, fish are caught using gigantic nets. For instance, the nets used by tuna fisherman (some are actually several miles wide) end up catching much more than just tuna. Estimates are that the average tuna net also traps up to 145 species of other fish, including manta rays, sharks, maki, sailfish, and king mackerel. These "nontargeted" fish are known as "bycatch" and don't hold any value to the fisherman. As a result, they're usually left on the deck of the ship to suffocate and are later tossed back into the ocean when they're dying or already dead.

Shrimping is the worst offender when it comes to bycatch. Shrimp live near the bottom of the sea, so they're caught using nets that are pulled along the ocean floor—where a lot of other creatures happen to live too. When shrimpers pull up their nets, 80 to 90 percent of what they've caught ends up being bycatch. The result is that for every pound of shrimp that's caught, twenty-six additional pounds of bycatch are killed in the process.

Across the board, the numbers are staggering when it comes to bycatch. Some experts have found that every year over sixty-three billion pounds of marine life are thrown back into the water as bycatch.

Keep all that needless suffering and waste in mind next time you think about having a tuna fish sandwich or some popcorn shrimp. As Foer puts it in *Eating Animals*, "Imagine being served a plate of sushi. But this plate holds all of the animals that were killed for your serving of sushi. The plate might have to be five feet across."

When you add up our seemingly insatiable appetite for fish like tuna, salmon, bass, and shrimp along with all the bycatch that are killed too, the result is that our oceans are in a very precarious state. According to the UN Food and Agriculture Organization, "over 70 percent of the world's fish species are either fully exploited or depleted." Some scientists say that if we don't stop commercial fishing, within fifty years the seas will largely be empty of fish.

Though it's getting a lot of hype, farm fishing isn't the answer either. You can't see it because it's happening under the water, but the conditions for farm-raised salmon are every bit as bad as they are for cows or pigs raised in a CAFO. According to PETA, despite being two and a half feet long, a salmon raised on an "aqua farm" spends its entire life in a space smaller than a bathtub. That's downright luxurious compared to the conditions farm-raised trout are forced to live in: twenty-seven full-grown fish packed into that same bathtub-size space.

The suffering of these fish is something I need to do a better job of staying conscious of. If there's one type of animal product I'm most likely to slip up and nibble a little piece of, it's definitely fish.

I know better, so I've got to do better. Just as I try to encourage my pescetarian friends to do just a little bit better too. If you can be just a fraction less harmful in your actions and give up fish, you're going to feel so much better about yourself!

WE HAVE DOMINION OVER ANIMALS!

> *"People often say that humans have always eaten animals, as if this is justification for continuing the practice. According to this logic, we should not try to prevent people from murdering other people, since this has also been done since the earliest of recorded times."* —ISAAC BASHEVIS SINGER

I've spoken about the horrors experienced by chickens, cows, pigs, and fish, but that's hardly the whole story when it comes to our abuse of animals. I haven't mentioned the three hundred million turkeys that are killed every year for their meat. Or the four million sheep. Or the estimated twenty million monkeys, mice, and rats killed every year for medical or product testing. Their suffering is almost unspeakable: monkeys having their heads slammed into walls at forty miles per hour to simulate car crashes. Restrained rabbits having chemicals injected into their eyes. (The pain is so immense that many literally break their backs trying to get out of their restraints.) Dogs having their heart rate increased to 240 times a minute for four to seven weeks until they die of heart attacks. When you read the stories—and especially see the pictures—of what happens to animals in these laboratories, it makes your stomach hurt and your heart ache.

"If you want to test cosmetics, why do it on some poor animal who hasn't done anything? They should use prisoners who have been convicted of murder or rape instead. So, rather than seeing if perfume irritates a bunny rabbit's eyes, they should throw it in Charles Manson's eyes and ask him if it hurts."

—Ellen DeGeneres

What makes it so easy for us to ignore all this cruelty and suffering even though its scale is so immense?

I believe one reason is there's a significant portion of the population that subscribes to the theory that humans have dominion over animals. I can talk all day about animals having their teeth ripped out with pliers, being starved of food and water, and being killed in a variety of barbaric ways, but the response will be, "That doesn't sound too nice, but the Bible does state we have dominion."

Sorry, but that's got to be one of the silliest things I've ever heard. I'm not much of a biblical scholar, but I refuse to believe that the Bible ever intended to cosign the industrialized system of suffering that we currently support. A king has dominion over his kingdom. Does that mean it's OK for him to torture and kill all his subjects? Of course not. Well, it's no different for our so-called dominion over the animals.

When the Bible spoke of dominion over the animals, it referred to watching over and protecting them. And yes, eating animals when necessary. But a shepherd killing several goats to feed his family and a

CAFO slaughtering millions of pigs every year have nothing in common. I have to believe that the authors of the Bible would be horrified if they saw how we kill the food we eat today.

Maybe you think I'm too much of a yogi to understand the Bible or even that I have an anti-Christian bias. If so, then consider these words from Matthew Scully, the Republican (and avowed Christian) speech writer I mentioned earlier, on why the whole dominion argument doesn't hold water:

> *Among its other wisdom about empathy for animals, Catholic teaching here advises: "We are bound to act toward them in a manner comfortable to their nature." And even in our secular age, one is hard put to think of any principle of Christian moral conduct so thoroughly or casually disregarded. That single injunction, were it actually applied, would go a long way toward ridding us of cruelty in general and especially of the factory farm.*

What really disturbs me about the dominion argument is it reflects a very dangerous pattern of using the Bible to justify some of humankind's worst actions. I'll go so far as to say if you're the type of Christian who believes CAFOs are justified by dominion, then you probably would have been the type of Christian who would have had interpreted the Bible as supporting slavery too.

I realize that's a comparison that will upset some people, but I'm not trying to suggest that human slaves were somehow equal to pigs. Stop it. Instead, I'm asking you to note the striking similarities in attitude and approach between slavery and CAFOs. Both are systems where maximizing profit trumps compassion and empathy. Both are systems that employ violence to get results. And the forces behind both have pointed to the Bible to try to make society think what they're doing is OK.

I'm not the only one who has noticed the parallels. The other day I was in a Rasta juice bar that had diagrams of slave ships up on the wall right next to their Ital (vegetarian) menus. To me, the message was crystal clear: Stop participating in unconscious behavior that is harmful to other beings. Behavior that will make you sick.

The editors of the *Vegan News* made the connection in their debut issue back in 1944 when they wrote, "We can see quite plainly that our present civilization is built on the exploitation of the animals, just as past civilizations were built on the exploitations of the slaves, and we believe the spiritual destiny of man is such that in time he will view with abhorrence the idea that men once fed on the products of animals' bodies."

> "If you want to know where you would have stood on slavery before the Civil War, don't look to where you stand on slavery today. Look to where you stand on animal rights."
>
> —Dr. Paul Watson of the *Sea Shepherd*

I don't make the slavery comparison lightly. Slavery is the system that stripped my ancestors of their pride and possessions and brought them to this country in chains. Slavery is the system that forced my ancestors to live without freedom and work without compensation for generations. Slavery is the system that created so many of the inequalities African Americans still encounter today. Understanding the horrific impact of slavery is why I agreed to be the Goodwill Ambassador for a UN memorial honoring the victims of the transatlantic slave trade. I wanted to do my part to ensure that something as devastating to the human condition as slavery will never happen again. Just as I want to ensure that something as devastating to both the human and the animal condition as eating animal products is ultimately judged just as harshly as slavery is today.

In the way I make comparisons between the meat industrial complex and slavery, others have made the same comparisons with Nazism. It can be a very unpopular parallel to draw—earlier in 2015, I got slammed by several Jewish groups after a few news outlets tried to suggest that I had compared the suffering of the horses that pull carriages around in Central Park to the Jewish victims of the Holocaust. While I did, and still do, abhor how those horses are treated, I never compared their situation to that of the victims of the Holocaust. Those headlines were concocted by reporters and editors who felt threatened by my actual statement: that the murder of billions of animals worldwide every year is a holocaust. The situation with the horses at Central Park might just be a small microcosm of a much larger problem, but that doesn't mean the larger problem doesn't exist.

Speaking of Singer, if you're not familiar, he was an iconic Jewish writer who grew up in a Warsaw ghetto and fled to America on the eve of the Holocaust. In his classic book *Enemies: A Love Story*, he describes the reaction of one of his characters, a Jewish survivor of the Holocaust, to watching an animal killed for its meat:

> *As often as Herman had witnessed the slaughter of animals and fish, he always had the same thought: in their behavior towards creatures, all men were Nazis. The smugness with which man could do with other species as he pleased exemplified the most extreme racist theories, the principle that might is right.*

Singer didn't write those words lightly—he was a European Jew who understood all too well just how cruel and inhumane the Nazi mentality was. Who spent most of his life trying to make sense of the damage the Nazis did to his family and his world. When he writes, "in their behavior towards creatures, all men were Nazis," you can feel the pain of that truth.

Notice that Singer didn't say that people are Nazis *all* the time, but rather just in how they treat animals. It's a crucial distinction and really gets to the heart of what I'm trying to convey in this section. Eating animals does not make you a terrible person. It does not make you a Nazi. Or a slave trader.

It does, however, represent some of our most unconscious behavior. Our unconscious mind that can make us blind to another being's suffering. That allows us to hold on to racist theories. That allows us to put our own perceived needs over the common good.

"The worst sin toward our fellow creatures is not to hate them, but to be indifferent to them: that's the essence of inhumanity."

—George Bernard Shaw

Breaking out of that sort of unconscious mind-set is why I go to yoga. Why I practice meditation. And yes, why I don't eat animal products.

As long as I'm participating in a system of abuse and suffering, I know I'll always be stuck. I'll always be a little sick spiritually (to say nothing of physically). I'll never reach my full potential.

I also know that as long as I eat animal products, history won't judge me kindly. We all like to believe we would have stood up to the proslavery voices if we had been alive during that era, or spoken out against Nazis if we had been around in prewar Germany. The truth is the majority of people at those times didn't. They simply went along with the program. We like to imagine ourselves as lions, bold creatures that don't follow the pack. But most of us act more like sheep, following along with something that might not feel right just because everyone else is doing it.

Fifty years from now, our grandchildren are going to ask, "Did Grandpa really eat animal products? That's so disgusting. Didn't it make him sick?" The same way that from a moral standpoint a kid today might be incredulous that one of his ancestors owned a restaurant with "colored" seating. Or that they didn't support women voting.

Don't have your grandkids or great-grandkids looking at you the way a kid today would look at segregationist. When they look back at you years from now, be seen in the same light as the abolitionists who fought against slavery, or as a protestor who spoke out against Hitler. Don't let history count you as one of the sheep who stayed quiet and looked the other way while people around them were being sold in chains or thrown in the ovens.

ANGRY VEGANS

"I got a right to be hostile. My people are being persecuted!"

—*PUBLIC ENEMY*

Before I close this section, I want to circle back and touch on the concept of the judgmental, or angry vegan, mentioned in the Misconceptions chapter.

Maybe you didn't get it then, but after having learned more about how we abuse animals, can you understand better now why some vegans might seem just a tad angry?

When your lenses are cleared and you can see what's truly happening in the meat and dairy industries, it's very hard to stay quiet about it. The question then becomes, just how loudly do you speak out?

It can be hard to find a balance. "If we're too graphic, people turn away," says Simone. "If we're too gentle, we don't make any impact." It's a balance I've struggled to find in my own life. As I said, in previous books I've held back a bit when talking about my decision to go vegan, especially regarding the abuse of the animals. I know it isn't a comfortable subject for most people and I've often chosen to take a softer, less confrontational approach than friends like Simone or Glen have.

Simone is still lying down on sidewalks naked and covered in blood to try to shock people into becoming more conscious about where the meat in the supermarket comes from. She still stands outside of Sea World and politely—but firmly—tries to talk to families about why they should reconsider supporting the exploitation of animals in captivity.

Glen's not out lying on sidewalks, but he's just as vocal in speaking out about the dangers of milk and dairy. For instance, Glen was one of the first people to ever photograph the skating legend Tony Hawk. So when he saw Hawk participated in the "Got Milk" campaign several years back, Glen sent Hawk a very blunt open letter asking him to reconsider his participation. "Do you realize what you are doing by allowing your good name and image to be used by the dairy council to promote milk? What kind of contract did they ask you to sign?" wrote Glen. "May I ask how much they paid you to participate in the campaign? Did you really need that money, or was it basically to promote your image? I don't mean to pick on you at all, by the way, I am just really curious. I would love to know these answers just because I'd like to know how the council protects itself with those that they ask to promote their products and how much they pay stars to sell their deadly foods."

They ended up having a little public back-and-forth on the issue, but ultimately Hawk respected Glen for standing up for his beliefs. Still, to some, Glen's approach probably epitomizes what they consider to be an angry vegan. I know Glen's approach might be antagonist or grating, but it will also wake people up. I like to compare it to the roles

Martin Luther King Jr. and Malcolm X played in the civil rights movement. (And no, I'm not even remotely comparing Glen and myself to Martin or Malcolm.)

Remember, if Malcolm X wasn't scaring the shit out of everyone talking about "by any means necessary" and refusing to back down, then King wouldn't have been as effective. If Malcolm X hadn't been on 125th Street calling the white man the devil and refusing to make any compromises, then King's path wouldn't have seemed like a better alternative to mainstream America. So even if you don't "need" an angry vegan attacking you for supporting dairy, reminding you of how you're ruining the planet, or throwing paint on a rich woman's fur coat, there's someone else out there who *does* need that wake-up call. Someone else who does need to be shocked out of their compliancy.

My approach has always been more "Martin" than "Malcolm." Maybe because I've been so unconscious in my own life, I'm not as quick to call people out and beat them over the head for their own ignorance. I'm more comfortable hoping that my own lifestyle and happiness will catch your attention. Woody Harrelson said something similar once when asked why he doesn't push his vegan lifestyle on his friends and acquaintances. "I try not to preach about diet anymore," he told a British newspaper. "I used to do that because I see so many people eating shit. Now I just let people see my energy and how strong I stay."

Sometimes a preachy and aggressive approach is required, though. Sometimes a message needs to be delivered that's so strong it will cut right through all the grit and grime that's accumulated on your lenses over the years. This is why I want to suggest several videos for you or for any of your friends who might need a wake-up call to watch.

I can talk about the conditions in these CAFOs all day, but the truth is I'm not nearly a good enough writer to even begin to fully convey the levels of brutality and suffering that goes on in those facilities.

The following videos do convey it. In very unflinching terms.

Start by watching *Diet for a New America*. It's almost twenty-five years old by this point, but it's still going to smack you across the face the way it woke me up years ago.

Then watch *Forks over Knives*, which I've already mentioned. It unflinchingly describes the incredible damage the meat and dairy industries are doing to both our bodies and our world. Katy Perry and the comedian Russell Brand watched it together when they were married and afterward Russell said that the movie motivated him to become a vegan. Oprah called it "provocative documentary" and Dr. Oz said, "I loved it and I need all of you to see it."

Finally, please watch a movie called *Earthlings*. If the other films didn't get to you, this one is going to hit you right in the gut. There's simply no way that you can watch this film and not be shook down to your foundation.

I can write about pigs being thrown into pens so cramped that they suffocate, but to actually see it happening will devastate you. When you actually see a piglet being castrated, you're going to turn away in horror. When you actually see a worker rub tobacco in a downer cow's eye in order to make it stand up, it's going to move you out of your unconscious state once and for all. Ellen DeGeneres watched it and said she could never look at meat the same again. I'll let her have the final word:

I have to tell you, Earthlings *is hard to watch. It took me a while, but I finally forced myself to watch it because I wanted to educate myself instead of being ignorant to the reality of it.*

What I learned is ignorance is not bliss. Ignorance is ignorance. You can't help or contribute to this planet without knowing what's really going on.

I became a vegan because I love animals, but also because I care about the planet and my health, and right now the way we are creating our food is hurting both. If you care about what you're putting in your body and feeding your family, you should watch Earthlings. *It changed my life.*

HOW TO DO IT

Congratulations! Learning the truth about the animals we eat and how it affects the world isn't the easiest information to, ahem, digest.

A lot of people are much more comfortable putting down a book like this and returning to their unconscious state than addressing it head-on.

But not you.

You've made it this far because you do want to make a healthier choice. A more sustainable choice. A more compassionate choice.

Those are some of the most beautiful choices you can make in your time here on earth, so please enter into this transformative stage of your life with an open and happy heart. You should feel great about what's to come.

As we've discussed, there are inevitably going to be some people in your family or your circle who aren't going to be as excited about your decision. Who are going to wonder, often aloud, if what you are about to do is too hard. Too restrictive.

It's not. As you'll see, a plant-based diet is far more varied and diverse than most people expect. If anything, you're going to find that your food choices and flavor experiences are more diverse than when you were eating animal products.

The meat and dairy industries have limited our choices, narrowed our tastes, and taken away our true food traditions. When we go to the supermarket, what we find are generally limited to items that can be shipped without getting damaged and aren't easily perishable. In other words, a lot of items in boxes or wrapped in plastic.

Those are the items that are going to keep you stuck in a bad place. Or even accelerate your decline. But plants don't come in a box or wrapped in plastic. Vegetables and fruit are fresh, which is how you were designed to eat food. It's great to base your diet on food that actually goes bad in a few days. Eating a lot of food that could go bad is probably the best sign that you're doing something *right*.

In this chapter I'm going to start by discussing how to set realistic goals when embarking on this journey. Goals to set you up for success rather than self-doubt or disappointment.

I'm also going to share some helpful tips on what new foods you should be buying for your kitchen and how to prepare them—and what foods you should be getting rid of. And it's not just meats and dairy! I'll also give you tips for ordering from restaurants, going to parties, and grabbing snacks when you're on the go.

Speaking of communication, I'll also share some tactics on how to talk with your friends who don't understand what you're doing. Or openly don't approve of it. Their disapproval can become a bigger barrier than you might think, but with the right approach it won't trip you up!

SET YOUR OWN SCHEDULE, BUT STICK TO IT!

When it comes to embarking on your journey toward a happy and healthier lifestyle, I promote a gradual—and flexible—approach. I believe an approach rooted in flexibility, instead of absolutism, is the one that will *keep* you vegan. Ultimately, that is what's most important.

Even my friends who are very strict vegans today didn't go cold turkey when they first made the switch. They followed a path that made the most sense for them. "I first cut out beef and chicken," recalls Glen. "Then about two months later I cut out fish, which I only ate a few times a month anyway. Maybe about a year after the first steps, I cut out all dairy." Glen adds that his transition might have been a bit faster if today's food options had been available to him. "Back in 1987 it was *waaaay* more difficult," he says. "No substitutes for most animal products were available at that time, no fake cheeses or meats were to be found, it was all tofu, beans, rice, and fruits and vegetables."

Personally, my evolution took about a year too. I didn't turn off *Diet for New America*, say "That's it!" and never take a bite of meat or dairy again. Instead, I started by giving up red meat while I was still on vacation in St. Barts. I didn't find it too hard; it got even easier once I realized how much more energy and clarity I had once I wasn't stuffing hamburgers down my throat all the time.

Buoyed by my experience with giving up beef, about a month later I decided to give up pork too. Outside of bacon and my morning sausage sandwich with jelly, I didn't really eat it too much. I still could eat eggs when I was grabbing breakfast or chicken if I was out at a restaurant. I continued on that path for a few more months, but the idea of all those chickens suffering on my behalf kept gnawing at me. I knew it was time for the next step and gave up chicken and eggs and fish, which essentially made me a vegetarian.

As I mentioned earlier, my transition from vegetarian to vegan was really kick-started by hearing my yoga teacher Dechen Thurman say at the end of class, "Now go out there and put something into your body that fuels your practice and makes it better. Not slows it down."

The idea of clogging up all that free-flowing energy I'd experienced in class didn't sit right with me. Of course meat was out of the question, but I started to realize that dairy wasn't enhancing my practice either. Drinking a green juice or eating a salad would enhance my practice. Drinking dairy or eating cheese was going to do the opposite.

Not long after that class I gave up dairy—milk, cheese, yogurt— and I've tried to practice a vegan diet religiously ever since.

Yet even though I promote a gradual approach, I'm still not a big fan of programs like Meatless Mondays, where people commit themselves to not eating any meat on Mondays. Or Vegan Before Six, in which you eat meat only for dinner. Don't get me wrong—Meatless Monday and Vegan Before Six can be great places to start if they feel accessible or attractive to you. But they should never become your destination. The goal is to cause the *least* harm, not just *less* harm. As Simone likes to say, feeling good about not eating meat once a week is like a slave owner wanting a pat on the back for giving his slaves Mondays off. You might be enlightened for a slave owner, but what's that really saying? You're still part of the problem.

Instead of adopting a program like Meatless Monday, when you feel like you're ready to give up animal products, make a commitment to that process and then stick to it. I've found that it helps to not just make that commitment to yourself but to your family and friends too. Let everyone know that at the start of the next month, you're going to stop eating beef. Whether they support that decision or not. And then talk about it until you almost have no choice but to live up to your word.

That's how I kicked drugs. When my lifestyle had become too much, toward the end of the year I started telling everyone that I was going to start living clean on January 1. I told my girlfriend, my friends, my coworkers, and my family. I talked about it so much that I would have looked like a goddammed fool if someone had seen me getting high on January 2.

What I'm asking you to do in this book is sooooooo much easier than giving up drugs. Hard drugs are a physical addiction. I promise you, this is nothing like that.

All I'm asking you to do is change your routine. That's it. Which is something you have already proven you can do. If you move to a new city, you have to change your routine. If you get a new job, you have to change your routine. If you have kid, it's time to change your routine.

Giving up animal products is just another change to your routine. It might feel a little strange at first, but you'll get used to it. So rather than spend months agonizing over when to start, just pick a day to give up meat and then stick to it. It's really that easy.

At that point you'll be a bona fide vegetarian, which is a major accomplishment! Be very proud of yourself. Please don't, however, end your journey. Remember what I wrote about the terrible conditions dairy cows are kept in before they are brutally slaughtered. Don't forget the damage consuming dairy does to your circulation and how it worsens allergies and respiratory problems. Don't forget about all the research linking it to various types of cancer.

As you begin the transition from vegetarian to vegan, one of the most helpful things you can do is to begin to experiment with the various dairy substitutes that are now available on the market. There are all sorts of soy-based milks, soy sour creams, soy cream cheeses, and soy ice creams available. For a long time those were essentially the only choices, but now there are cheeses and creams based on almond milk, coconut milk, hemp milk, and even rice milk. Try different ones out and see which ones are most appealing to your taste buds. Try a soy-based sour cream on your vegetarian chili, or have a bowl of almond milk ice cream. Figure out which tastes you enjoy and which ones don't work for you. That way when you decide it's time to fully transition to vegan, you'll be going into the process with the knowledge that there are dairy substitutes out there that are going to allow you to enjoy cheeses, ice cream, and milks without the harmfulness and suffering.

No matter what path you take toward veganism, you could have moments where you slip up or lose your way. Do not get discouraged if this happens. It doesn't make you a bad person who is insensitive to animals' plights. It doesn't make you a hypocrite. It just makes you a human who's still working on your evolution. There's zero shame in that.

I've said that I practice veganism religiously, but there have been plenty of moments where I lose that religion. I'm prone to sneaking in a chicken here or a piece of fish there, if I think nobody is listening. Just like I'll order the egg noodle soup every now and then. When those moments happen, however, I won't get down on myself and fall off the vegan wagon.

Instead, I say sorry to any animals I have harmed, forgive myself for having given in to an urge that wasn't helpful, and then recommit myself to the practice of eating and living compassionately.

There have been times where I've actually give myself permission to cheat. During my most recent trip to St. Barts I thought, "Screw it. I'm getting a chicken burger the next time I'm at JoJo's. It's not going to be the end of the world." But when I sat down at JoJo's and looked at the menu, there was the veggie burger listed right next to the chicken burger. I already knew the veggie was delicious, plus it didn't come with a side of suffering. Why would I bring all that negativity into my life? For three minutes of selfish "pleasure"? Especially when I knew the chicken burger wasn't any better than that delectable veggie burger? So I made the compassionate choice and enjoyed the hell out of that veggie burger.

People have different ways of dealing with the desire to cheat. I know one guy who will eat oysters or mussels if he's feeling a strong craving for a nonvegan meal. His rationale is that oysters and mussels don't have central nervous systems, so they probably don't feel any pain when they're killed. A lot of vegans wouldn't accept that reasoning, but it works for him. After a dozen or so oysters, he's ready to go back to his all-vegan diet.

Beyoncé's nutritionist, Marco Borges, said that even while promoting her vegan challenge, Bey still ate "a little fish here and there." Venus Williams even coined a term—*chegan*—for her nonabsolutist version of a plant-based diet. "If it's on your plate, I might get to cheat.

If you're sitting next to me, good luck. You turn your head once and your food might be gone," Venus told CBS. "I'm not perfect, so I forgive myself when I make mistakes and I do a lot of juicing as well."

Venus's approach is very practical because it can become very easy to beat yourself up for your mistakes. Some people are so freaked out by the idea of cheating on their diets that it seems easier to isolate themselves from the world. That's what happened to André 3000 of the rap group OutKast after he went vegan. "I was kind of just sitting at home eating a salad," he told *Esquire*. "You become mean. That's not good for you. Sometimes when you're trying too hard to follow a rule, you're doing yourself more harm."

André's right—you don't want to give up animal products just to become someone who's so rigid about being a vegan that it overshadows everything else in your life. You also don't want to become that vegan whose judgmental attitude keeps other people inside their houses. If someone tells you they're vegan, but then you catch them sneaking a piece of fish at a party, don't give that moment any weight. You don't know that person's situation or their heart. It could be the first piece of fish she's had in twenty-five years, or it could be the twenty-fifth piece she's had that week. Instead of going out of your way to criticize such people, go out of your way to support them. With love, remind them that the hummus tastes really great. Help remind them that no matter how bad, or how often, they've stumbled, the best thing they can do is stay on their path.

EATING AS YOU EVOLVE

When transitioning into a vegan diet, it's not enough to only remove foods from you diet. You also have to begin to add new foods in. Otherwise you're going to become bored by your food options and eventually lose your appetite, as it were, for going vegan.

I have a good friend this happened to. He decided to give up meat and found that he didn't actually miss it that much at all. What he didn't do, however, was work on finding new plant-based dishes to replace the animal products. As a result, he ended up eating a lot of pastas, breads, and cereals. He quickly gained a lot of weight—the carbs in pasta will do that to you—and also became bored with his suddenly limited diet. After a few months of living that way he told me that going vegan "wasn't working for him" and he was going to start eating meat again. But when I asked him what wasn't working, it became apparent his problem wasn't giving up animal products; he just hadn't figured out the right things to replace them with.

Remember, being vegan isn't just about cutting out animal products. It's just as much about building plant-based foods into your diet. The kind of foods that are going to be better for you and better for the environment. So let's check out some of the foods you should start incorporating into your meals.

Leafy Greens

Leafy green vegetables should be the foundation of your plant-based diet. These are the plants that are going to give you all the protein you need now that you're not eating animal products. Plus, since they are filled with fiber and vitamins, they are going to give you more energy and help boost your immune system. They're also rich with antioxidants, which means they'll decrease your risk for certain cancers and cardiovascular disease.

Bok choy	**Iceberg lettuce**	**Spinach**
Broccoli	**Kale**	**Swiss chard**
Cabbage	**Mustard greens**	**Turnip greens**
Dandelion greens	**Romaine lettuce**	

If you see a green vegetable at the grocery store or farmers' market, don't be intimidated. Try it! Rule of thumb is that green vegetables always taste good sautéed with garlic.

Whether you eat them sautéed, in salads, soups, stir-fries, or just raw, you want to incorporate as much of these greens into your diet as possible. If I'm at home and need a quick bite to eat, I'll just sauté a little spinach with garlic and put some hot sauce on it. It takes less than five minutes to make and always fills me up.

Another way I try to make sure I'm always getting enough leafy greens is through juicing. Every day—morning, noon, and night, if I can help it—I drink a green juice, which includes kale, parsley, spinach, cucumber, and apple. Not only is it healthy but it gives me the same kind of high I feel after I meditate. I get my juices cold-pressed from a shop in L.A. called Clover and from Juice Press when I'm in NYC. But that might not be an option for everyone. Good juice places can be hard to find and are often pretty expensive when you do.

Instead, try juicing at home. You'll want to invest in a good juicer, which can run a couple hundred dollars, but you'll save a lot of money in the long run. One thing you want to watch when juicing, however, is your sugar intake. Because it removes fiber, juicing concentrates the sugar that's naturally in fruits and vegetables. Apples, beets, and carrots in particular all contain a lot of sugar, so be conscious of how much of them you incorporate into your juices.

Beans and Legumes

Along with leafy greens, beans and legumes should be the other pillar of your vegan diet. Not only are they cheap, but they're also filled with nutrients. According to the FDA, a single half-cup serving of legumes or beans will provide you with 15 percent of your daily recommended protein, 20 percent of your recommended fiber, and 24 percent of your recommended folic acid.

If you're not familiar with the term, *legume* simply refers to any plant that carries its fruit inside a pod. There are over eighteen thousand types of legumes, but some of the best known ones are green peas, snap peas, fava beans, kidney beans, edamame, soy nuts, peanuts, lima beans, and lentils.

There are hundreds of great bean dishes out there, including bean burritos, salads, chili, casseroles, soups, and even breads. When I was on Dr. Oz's show one time, the famed New Orleans chef Emeril Lagasse showed us how to make a white bean and Tuscan kale stew that blew us away. As Dr. Oz pointed out, it not only was filled with nutrients but was also incredibly tasty.

I encourage you to experiment with lentil-based dishes. Lentils are among the healthiest (and cheapest) foods in the world, and their benefits include helping lower cholesterol, aid digestion, and increase energy. Lentil loaf is a great substitute for meat loaf, lentil and brown rice burgers are a great replacement for hamburgers, and I find lentil soups to be incredibly hearty. I'll usually have a lentil soup for lunch a couple of times a week, and curried lentils (dal) are among my favorite dishes when I eat at Indian restaurants.

Protein and B$_{12}$

One of the things you'll hear a lot when you start your evolution are warnings that you won't get enough protein when you cut animal products out of your diet.

You might even have some very well-meaning people come up to you and say something like, "I know you want to change your diet, but I'm really concerned about where you're getting your protein from if you do that."

While that person undoubtedly has your best interest at heart, there really isn't that much for him to worry about. While we all need to consume a certain amount of protein to be healthy, the fact is that those levels are very easy to achieve without eating animal products.

"As protein sources, beans and nuts have some advantages over animal sources. They give you fiber, vitamins, minerals, and healthy unsaturated fats. Like fruits and vegetables, they also give you a host of phytochemicals, an ever-expanding collection of plant products that help protect you from a variety of chronic diseases."

—Dr. Walter Willett, Harvard School of Public Health

If anything, that well-meaning friend would be better off giving warnings to someone who *does* eat animal products. That's because most Americans eat two to six times the amount of protein that's nutritionally recommended anyways.

Mark Bittman, the *New York Times* reporter and best-selling author, calls this perception the "protein myth." "The average American eats two to three times as much protein as he or she needs," Bittman tells *Men's Fitness* magazine. "The 'myth' I've labeled is multilayered: Americans have been urged by food marketers to consume far more animal products than we should be eating, and many people don't realize that there's plenty of protein in plants. In fact, many plants have more protein per calorie than meat. While meat, eggs, and cheese are, sure, nutrient-dense, they're calorie-dense too, and they're usually produced in, let's say, not-ideal conditions. Plants provide the same vitamins and minerals plus protein—along with phytonutrients not found in meat."

Steve Wynn, the billionaire hotel and restaurant magnate who became a vegan several years ago, is even more blunt about this country's misinformed views on protein and meat. "The notion that you need animal food as protein is one of the great conspiracies of bullshit by the government," says Wynn, who recently opened up the Viva Las Vegan restaurant in one of his casinos. "Did we not all grow up saying we had to have four glasses of whole milk a day for healthy bones? It's ridiculous. It's liquid cholesterol."

Steve's right, don't let them trick you into thinking that you can't get the protein you need if you go vegan. Former NFL star Ricky Williams says he managed to get more than enough protein while playing in the league by eating veggies, quinoa, hemp, beans, seeds, nuts, and vegan shakes.

And those are just some of the options. Check out this list of other great sources of protein:

Almond butter	Chickpeas	Peas
Almonds	Coconuts	Pecans
Avocado	Collard greens	Pinto beans
Bean sprouts	Hemp seeds	Seitan
Black-eyed peas	Kale	Soy milk
Broccoli	Kidney beans	Sunflower seeds
Brown rice	Lima beans	Swiss chard
Brussels sprouts	Macadamia nuts	Tahini
Bulgur	Oatmeal	Tempeh
Cauliflower	Pasta	Tofu
Chia	Peanut butter	Walnuts

Personally, I make sure I eat plenty of beans, chickpeas, peas, and lentils. I've found they give me more than enough protein, and I've never suffered from any feeling that I somehow didn't have enough energy or strength. If anything, my energy and sense of strength have largely increased since I gave up animal products.

Now, while the idea that you need to closely watch your protein intake after giving up meat is largely a myth, you do have to be careful in monitoring your vitamin B_{12} levels. B_{12} is an essential vitamin we get mainly from meat, dairy, and fish. Your body stores excess B_{12} in its liver, but when you stop eating those foods, the store becomes depleted over time. When you do run out of B_{12}, it can make you pretty sick. It can start with headaches and fatigue and lead to neurological and nerve damage if it's not treated.

Vitamin B_{12} deficiency can be scary, but it's also easily avoidable. When you do make the decision to cut meat out of your diet, go see your doctor and get your blood work done. If you tend to be low on B_{12}, you'll probably get a shot. If not, you can start taking supplements proactively so that you'll never develop an issue. Be diligent, but as Dr. Oz says of the B_{12} issue for vegans, "That's a little pill under your mouth every once and a while. Not a big deal."

Grains

As mentioned, grains will be a great source of protein and fiber in your diet. Though grains come in many varieties, you want to focus on whole grains, such as quinoa (great for people with gluten allergies), buckwheat, barley, brown rice (also gluten free), rye, spelt, and oats.

Quinoa (pronounced *keen-wa*), an ancient grain from South

America that was the food staple of the Inca empire, has become especially popular in recent years because of its high levels of protein, calcium, magnesium, and manganese. Cooked quinoa has a fluffy yet crunchy texture that people enjoy and is great for use in salads or for breakfast. I enjoy quinoa in salads with cranberries and cashews or with blueberries for breakfast.

Whenever possible, avoid refined grains like white flour, white rice, and white bread. Basically, if it's white, that means it's not all right. The problem is that those grains have been milled in a way that removes the germ and bran from the grain. It's done to improve texture and shelf life, but it also removes most of the nutrients.

One tip when reading the packaging on your bread (something you should get in the habit of doing with all the food you buy): Make sure it says "100% whole wheat," as opposed to just "100% wheat." If it's the latter, chances are it's refined. Also, any words like *enriched* and *bleached* are also giveaways that you're dealing with a refined grain. That also goes for pasta, where you want either whole wheat or semolina in Italian types like spaghetti, fettuccini, penne, and rigatoni.

If you have a gluten allergy, try Asian noodles like soba, a Japanese noodle made from buckwheat; dang myun, a Korean noodle made from sweet potato; or rice vermicelli, a noodle that's popular in Vietnam and other parts of Southeast Asia.

Nuts and Seeds

Nuts are going to become one of your go-to food sources, especially when it's time to snack. Nuts, especially tree nuts like almonds, cashews, and walnuts, are a fantastic source of healthy omega-3 fatty acids and have been linked to reduced cholesterol levels and inflammation, and increased weight loss. As a rule, Americans don't eat enough of them. "That may be because people are afraid of the fat and calories in nuts, or they find plain nuts boring," says Joy Bauer, a best-selling author and nutritionist who you've probably seen on the *Today* show. "That's a shame, because a small handful can pack your diet with filling protein, fiber, unsaturated fats, and important vitamins and minerals."

Embrace nut spreads like peanut butter, almond butter, hemp seed butter, and hazelnut butter. These spreads bring a lot of flavor and texture to your diet, and you can save a lot of money by making many of them at home. All you need is a food processor and your pick of flavors—coconut oil, cinnamon, vanilla, cacao powder, etc.—and you can make a really yummy nut spread in your kitchen from virtually any nut or seed.

Since nuts fill you up, throw a couple in a sandwich bag every morning and carry them around with you. They're perfect for a quick snack, especially if you feel low on energy during the late afternoon. Ground up, they are perfect as toppings on salads and vegetables.

Make sure to stock up on sunflower seeds, which make a great snack. Also look for recipes that include pumpkin seeds, sesame seeds, and flaxseeds, all of which are a tasty source of nutrients.

Fruit

Make sure you eat fruit at least a couple of times a day. Try to buy raw fresh fruit when possible, but if you have to get canned or dried fruit, that's better than not eating any at all. Even though I'm a proponent of juicing, it shouldn't be your only source of fruit (or vegetables for that matter), because it removes the fiber.

Make sure that every day you have at least one fruit that is high in vitamin C, like citruses, melons, and strawberries. Blueberries, cranberries, and blackberries should also be a big part of your diet. Dr. Oz carries a container of blueberries with him every single day because they're so rich in antioxidants, which reduce inflammation, support the immune system, and slow down the aging process.

Since many fruits—like strawberries, peaches, blueberries, and apples—are heavily sprayed with pesticides, this is one area where you're going to want to spend some extra money and buy organic.

There have been some suggestions that a vegan diet high in fruit could lead to increased tooth decay, but the studies on this have been inconclusive. However, it is true that fruit naturally has high sugar and acid levels, both of which aren't great for teeth. To be safe, rinse your mouth out with water after you eat fruit, especially those particularly high in sugar like apples and strawberries. The water will wash away most of the sugar and acid that might otherwise harm your teeth's enamel.

Root Vegetables

Root vegetables like carrots, beets, turnips, parsnips, and rutabagas are some of the healthiest foods you eat. Potatoes are great too until you load them up with butter and creams. On a vegan diet, you won't make that mistake. Instead, you'll get to enjoy all the benefits of potatoes—which include lots of vitamin C and fiber and low cholesterol—without any of the adverse effects of dairy.

Experiment with russet for baking, red and Yukon for sautéing, and sweet potatoes for roasting (note that if you are prediabetic or diabetic, sweet potatoes are the healthier choice because they don't add to your glycemic load). Also, most of the potato's nutrients are found under its skin, so make sure to leave that on no matter what dish you cook.

Spices and Seasonings

This is the most exciting part of being a vegan: welcoming new flavors into your life, exploring ways other cultures traditionally flavor their foods, and rediscovering your own heritage through herbs and spices. Reclaim what has been removed from your kitchen over the course of time and by the corporatization of our food system.

Why do people find themselves craving dairy and meat? Not because they somehow inherently taste better than vegetables, grains, or fruits but because people become addicted to dairy and meats high in fat, salt, and sugars. I've written about this before, but it bears repeating: That addiction is not an accident. The big meat distributors, especially the ones that sell processed meats, have spent tens of millions of dollars finding ways to make their products even saltier, fattier, and sweeter so that consumers will keep buying them. No matter how terrible those products are for their health.

If you've been a longtime consumer of animal products, your taste buds have been dulled to the point that they'll probably recognize only very high levels of salt, fat, and sugar. So as you begin your vegan evolution, it's critical that you experiment with different spices and seasonings in your cooking. By introducing new flavors and sensations to your diet, you'll ensure that you are adding good fats, sugars, and proteins. You're also going to wake up those taste buds that have been stuck in a processed-food rut for too long and introduce them to the wonderful flavors that come from cooking with a variety of seasonings and spices.

The first thing you'll want to do is make sure that you're well supplied with some basic herbs like basil, mint, thyme, oregano, rosemary, sage, dill, and parsley. Buying dried herbs is fine, but also try growing some of your own. Basil and mint in particular are very easy to grow in a little pot on your windowsill. The flavor you get from fresh herbs is fantastic, plus planting and watching herbs grow is a fun project to do with your kids.

After you're well stocked with the basics, ask yourself what types of cuisines you think you'll be cooking the most. If you're into Italian food, get some fennel, red pepper flakes, and garlic powder.

If you're into Asian foods, you'll want plenty of cumin, cardamom, mustard seeds, star anise, and Chinese five-spice powder. You'll also want condiments like soy sauce (make sure it's low sodium), rice vinegar, chili sauce, and sesame oil.

For Indian food, you'll want spices like turmeric, curry powder, green and black cardamom, cloves, cinnamon, and black peppercorn, plus ginger, cilantro, and tamarind paste.

There are wonderful Mexican options out there—vegan enchiladas, tacos, chilies, and tamales. To cook them, make sure you stock up on chili powder, cinnamon, cloves epazote, achiote paste, and mole rubs. Canned refried beans are also an inexpensive but filling option to keep around the house.

No matter what style you cook in, you'll also want to have several essential oils on hand: olive, coconut, flaxseed, corn, sunflower, safflower, sesame, and grapeseed, plus nut oils like peanut, hazelnut, and pine seed. Throw out any sprays or spreads that contain hydrogenated oils. Those are heavy on trans fats that lead to high cholesterol levels.

Whatever type of dish or taste you're looking for, there is likely a vegan version of it out there. From your grandmother's meatballs to your mother's chicken casserole, if you type the name of the dish plus the word *vegan* into Google, you're going to find plenty of options. I even found a couple great ones for my mother's spicy spaghetti and sausage.

Homemade dips and sauces will also enhance anything you are making. With a small food processor you can easily make pesto with basil, a clove of garlic, olive oil, cashews, and a little bit of lemon juice. This can keep for a few days in the fridge and you can spread it on whole wheat toast as a snack or mix it into whole wheat or semolina pasta, sautéed vegetables, or tofu. Experiment with different nuts, fresh green herbs like parsley and cilantro, jalapeño peppers, and coconut milk to make different sauces. Explore your own sense of taste!

The key is to have fun and experiment with all these different spices, oils, and condiments. Instead of bemoaning the meat and dairy dishes you can't have, celebrate the fact that you've finally been liberated from the salt-sugar-fat jail, and you can now enjoy such a wide range of flavors.

Milks and Cheeses

Just because you've stopped consuming dairy doesn't mean you can't have a bowl of cereal and milk in the morning. It just won't be cow's milk. That's not a problem, because there is a wide variety of plant-based milks you can replace that dairy with. Probably the most popular is soy milk, which has a creamy, smooth taste that some find reminiscent of dairy. My personal favorite is almond milk, which is a little nuttier but really grew on me. Other options include hemp milk, coconut milk, oat milk, rice milk, and hazelnut milk. Try them all out and learn which ones you like best. You might like almond milk in your cereal, but coconut milk in your coffee. Or if you're just looking for a treat, maybe you want a glass of hazelnut milk. The more familiar you become with the various flavors and textures, the less you'll miss cow's milk.

The other cool thing about milks is that they're very easy to make at home. You can find plenty of recipes online, but most of them involve soaking the nuts overnight, draining them, and then mixing them with fresh water in a blender. You can also enhance the flavor by adding dates, cinnamon, and/or vanilla extract, depending on your tastes. Making these milks at home will not only likely save you money but will also allow you to cut down on the high sugar level that's found in many of the brands sold in stores.

Giving up cheese is a hurdle a lot of people worry about, but it's not nearly as big a hurdle as you might think. Personally, I love a company called Daiya, which makes all sorts of wonderful cheese alternatives that don't contain dairy or soy. They've got shreds, wedges, slices, cream cheese–style spreads. Throw some of their shredded cheese on a pizza and you'll be straight.

You can also get vegan blue cheese, vegan brie, vegan feta, vegan goat cheese, even vegan mozzarella cheese that actually browns and stretches when you heat it. Most of the cheeses are made from plant products like soy protein, solidified vegetable oils, tapioca flour, and natural enzymes.

I'm even working with Beyond Meat, a company that uses thousands of different kinds of plants to come up with delicious meat alternatives. They use the same combination of amino acids, fats, carbohydrates, minerals, and water that gives meat its familiar chew, resistance, and variation, and create it from plants instead. They've already got a bunch of great "beef" and "chicken" products—my favorite is their meatballs with peppers, vegan cheese, and tomato sauce.

I'm also incredibly inspired by VBites Foods, a vegan food company that was started by Heather Mills, the environmental activist who was once married to Paul McCartney. VBites is the biggest vegan food supplier in the U.K. and has proven just how popular great vegan food can be.

If we can convince people to buy their meatballs from Beyond Meat, or their meat-free chorizo chunks from a company like VBites, think of how much good that would do. Replacing animal products with plant products will not only help people get healthier (for instance, none of VBites's products contain cholesterol) but also help save animals and the environment. Once consumers realize they can enjoy the tastes they're used to without having to harm animals, it's going to spell the end of factory farming. Just like horses didn't have to pull carriages once the car was invented, cows won't have to give up their bodies for hamburgers once we find the best plant alternative.

In a decade, we could be looking at the end of animal farming. I'm hopeful that, in time, the steps that Beyond Meat and others are taking today will result in nothing short of a food revolution.

Soy

I saved soy for last, even though it is the food most heavily associated with a vegan diet. Soy comes in many forms: raw as edamame or a nut, processed as tofu, or fermented as miso or tempeh. Many of the vegan dishes you'll order in a vegan restaurant or cook at home will use one of these soy products as meat substitutes.

Soy has many positive properties. Besides being wonderfully adaptable and able to mimic a lot of the textures and flavors of meat, soy will also provide you with plenty of protein. It also contains all eight essential amino acids. Studies have shown that soy might help prevent osteoporosis in women.

Tofu is the most popular form of soy, and you can make it easily at home. All it involves is heating soy milk with water, letting it curdle, and then pressing it into blocks. After letting the soybeans soak overnight, the entire process doesn't take more than a couple of hours.

Despite the simplicity in making it (it's been made in homes in Asia for thousands of years) there are some who have attacked tofu for being unhealthy because it's a processed food. That's technically true, but if you check the label on any tofu container (especially an organic brand) you'll see that the only ingredients are soybeans, water, and gypsum (a sulfate mineral that aids in curding). That's really not that bad, especially compared to most processed foods, which have probably more than twenty ingredients on the label, most of which are chemicals you can't even pronounce.

There's a growing belief in the vegan community that a lot of the negative information you read about soy products in general have been planted or funded by the dairy industry. I can't prove that, but I wouldn't put it past them either. After all, for every person who starts buying soy milk or choosing soy yogurt, that's someone not buying the dairy industry's products. And we all know the lengths they're willing to go to for profit.

It is true that as you evolve out of your old eating habits, you don't want to rely on soy-based processed foods too heavily. You'll get the most out of a plant-based diet when you're eating whole vegetables instead of ones that have been processed. But I also feel that for people who have spent their lives eating meat, it's inevitable that they're going to want foods that are in sync with their history when it comes to flavor and taste. If soy products like Chik'n Nuggets (my personal soft spot) or Tofurky or Smart Sausages can help ease someone's transition away from meat, then that's certainly better than the alternative. Should you base your diet around faux meat products made out of soy? Definitely not. But I take offense when some people label them as "vegan junk food." Because they're so much better for you than eating the real junk food you get in a fast-food restaurant.

Of course there is real junk food that also happens to be vegan. Food that, as PETA calls it, is "accidental vegan." Cap'n' Crunch Peanut Butter Crunch is technically vegan. So are Doritos spicy sweet chili-flavored tortilla chips. As are Fritos, Oreos, and graham crackers. As well as Kool-Aid and many energy drinks.

I'd certainly rather you snack on some Doritos than eat some chicken wings, but try to stay away from accidental vegan food as much as possible. Your focus should be on incorporating as many whole foods—foods that only have one ingredient—into your diet. For example, blueberries are a whole food. Blueberry *muffins* are processed. Potatoes are a whole food, potato *chips* are processed. Cashews are a whole food, cashew *energy bars* are processed.

Whenever possible, make your choice a whole choice. But if you slip up and snack on a few potato chips or have a bowl of sugary cereal for breakfast instead of oatmeal, remember it's not the end of the world. This book is called *The Happy Vegan* for a reason. As long as you're steadily moving toward a more healthy and compassionate lifestyle, you should always feel good about your food choices. Whether it's vegan junk food or accidental vegan, it's always a better choice than the animal alternative.

SOURCING YOUR FOOD

To get the most out of being a vegan, you'll want to cook at home as much as possible. There are a lot of benefits to this. It's much cheaper than ordering out, especially now that you're not buying animal products. You're going to love how your grocery bills look when you're mainly buying only vegetables, fruits, and grains (even if you buy organic). Cooking at home will also force you to play around with all those new spices and flavors, expanding your taste buds. And as discussed, cooking at home helps you lose weight. No matter how much sugar you might put into a dish, it's not going to be as much as a restaurant puts in. No matter how big a portion you serve yourself, chances are it won't be as large as the one you'd get in a restaurant.

All that home cooking means you're going to have to become a more thoughtful and savvy shopper. If you do most of your shopping in supermarkets, keep in mind that the healthiest products (veggies and fruits) are usually found along the periphery of the store, while the center aisles are where the heavily processed foods are. Within those center aisles, the most alluring products—those with the highest amounts of salt, sugar, and fat—are strategically placed at eye level. Healthier options are usually found on the lower or higher shelves.

That means you're either going to get up on your tippy toes or bend down low to find the plain oatmeal. If you go shopping and find everything you're picking out is at eye level, then you might not be getting the most nutritious stuff.

Also, start to get in the habit of checking the ingredients before you buy anything that comes in a box or a plastic bag. The first thing a lot of people look at is what percentage of carbs or how many grams of sugar a product has, but that's not the most pertinent information. What you really should ask is, "What are these ingredients I'm about to put in my body?" Especially if you can't pronounce most of them. As the best-selling author Michael Pollan writes, "If you can't say it, don't eat it." Pollan also says that the fewer ingredients a product has, the more healthful it likely is. "Don't buy products with more than five ingredients," he advises.

Checking the label before you buy something is also going to allow you to avoid animal products you might not have expected to find. For instance, these are all fairly generic-sounding ingredients, but they actually all contain animal products.

Casein	Diacetyl
Casein hydrolysate	Lactalbumin
Caseinates (in all forms)	Phosphate
Lactose	Lactoferrin
Lactulose	Whey

Casein and caseinates in particular are ones to watch out for. Casein is the protein found in cow's milk and it's used as a binding agent in a lot of different kinds of foods that are labeled "dairy-free" or "gluten-free," especially some soy yogurts. It's so good at binding that it's also used in glue, concrete, fabrics, and plastics.

It's not surprising that many researchers believe that casein plays a major role in the link between dairy and cancer. "Our work showed the casein is the most relevant cancer promoter ever discovered," says Dr. T. Colin Campbell.

Casein is also dangerous because it has addictive qualities, which means it could be contributing to your craving dairy without you even knowing it. "Casein, one of the proteins in milk, crosses the blood–brain barrier and becomes something called casomorphins," says Victoria Moran, the author of *Main Street Vegan*. "Yes'm, that sounds a lot like morphine—because casomorphin is also an opioid. Nature designed it that way so young mammals would enjoy nursing, come back for more, and live to reproduce themselves."

Also keep an eye out for items that include gelatin, a protein from animal skin, tendons, ligaments, and bones in water. It's used as a thickener for fruit gelatins and puddings, as well as in candies, marshmallows, cakes, ice cream, and yogurts. Also beware of products using lecithins, a substance that can come from soy but also often comes from egg yolk. It's found in a lot of cocoa and cocoa butter products. If you're worried about a specific ingredient, the PETA website has a very helpful "Animal Ingredients List," which will show you what to avoid.

PETA also provides a list of vegan items that can be found in major supermarkets. It's a very useful tool when you're first looking to restock your kitchen after giving up animal products. A similar list can be found on the HappyCow website.

Since deciphering labels can be tricky (and tiresome), whenever possible try to shop at farmers' markets. Foods that are grown locally are always going to be fresher and as a result filled with more nutrients. It's also good to get in the habit of eating foods that are in season. Whenever you eat a fruit or vegetable that isn't in season where you live, that means it had to be trucked or flown in to your area, often from overseas. That's extra stress on the environment, stress that can be eliminated when you eat locally. Plus we already know how much better small, family-owned farms are for the environment than CAFOs. Let's support these family farms before there aren't any more left.

If you don't know where there's a farmers' market near you, go to localharvest.org and type in your zip code. It'll show you the closest one.

Of course the ultimate family-run farm is the one you can start in your own home. If you have a backyard, start a container garden and grow your own runner beans, sunflowers, sweet corn, and tomatoes. If you live in the city and don't have a backyard, you can still put some flowerpots on your porch steps, or even on a sunny fire escape, and grow your own herbs like basil and mint.

Encourage your friends and neighbors to start their own little gardens too. You can trade seeds, as well as advice and observations. And ultimately produce too. You'll love being part of a community that's built around a nurturing life.

ORDERING OUT

Whether it's going out for dinner with your friends, grabbing a quick bite on the way home from work, or catching a meal in a new city while you're traveling, a lot of people worry that eating out as a vegan is going to be a difficult experience. While it's true that your experience may vary depending on what city you're in, I'm confident you're going to be able to find more than enough options to keep you happy.

If you're in Los Angeles or New York City, enjoy your pick of incredible vegan options. I already told you about Crossroads and Veggie Grill in L.A., but I also love Native Foods Café and Elf Cafe. When I'm in New York, I try to stop by the Jivamuktea Café, where I always get the spicy tempeh salad and dal. Some of my other top spots include Gobo and the House of Vegetarian, where I get the curry wheat gluten (I like to say that's my new version of chitlins). I'll also stop by the Indian restaurant Curry in a Hurry, where I get the curry eggplant or the saag paneer, which they make special for me without the cheese. You'll also want to ask them to cook the dish without ghee, which is a clarified butter used in many Indian restaurants. Even if you're not a regular like I was at Curry in a Hurry, never be afraid or embarrassed to ask a restaurant to prepare a vegetarian or vegan version of a dish for you. You're paying for the dish. There's nothing crazy about asking for it to be prepared the way you prefer. A meat eater doesn't think twice about asking a steak to be cooked well done. You shouldn't think twice about asking your server not to put cheese on your salad.

In cities like Chicago, San Francisco, Philadelphia, Boston, and Austin, you shouldn't have any problem finding lots of great options.

If you're not sure where to go, HolyCow has a great search engine which will bring up every vegan or vegetarian restaurant in your area.

If you can't get on HolyCow, or in the unlikely event there aren't any vegan or vegetarian spots in your area, look for Chinese, Mexican, and Indian restaurants. Pretty much no matter where you are in this country, there should be one of them. You can always get a bean burrito at a Mexican place. Every Chinese restaurant has their version of Buddha's delight, which is a vegetarian dish. You're always going to be able to get lentils and rice at an Indian restaurant. At a sushi place you can order maki rolls with sweet potato and peanuts or avocado and cucumber.

Keep in mind that a lot of fast-food chains are starting to carry vegan and vegetarian options as well. Chipotle is the most vegan-friendly chain, as well as being GMO-free. Applebee's has a strawberry and avocado salad that you can ask them to hold the chicken from. Burger King offers its BK Veggie (though it does contain dairy). The Cheesecake Factory also has a veggie burger made with brown rice, farro, couscous, mushrooms, and black bean as well as a penne pasta with tossed veggies. Little Caesars and Papa John's use vegan dough and pizza sauce. Just ask them to hold the cheese when you order a pie and you'll be good to go. You can find a complete list of fast-food options on PETA's website.

If you think you're going to be somewhere with limited options— like in an airport or on a long drive on a thruway—plan ahead and pack some food. Nuts and dried fruit are always a great option. Or you can follow Dr. Oz's lead and pack a small jar with blueberries or strawberries. I'll also pack a small bottle of my favorite hot sauce with me when I'm going to be on the road. That way I know that even if I end up with just a plate of rice and beans, they're going to taste just the way I like them. There are very few dishes a good hot sauce can't cure.

No matter what sort of restaurant or deli or food kiosk you end up in, simply do the best that you can in the situation. That means figuring out what sort of parameters you're comfortable with. I know plenty of vegans who aren't willing to make any concessions. If there's even a chance a dish might have animal products in it, they're not going to touch it. You might find that too strict, but I'm inspired by their commitment. Even if I don't always match it.

It's true, I'm not quite as restrictive. If I find out something was cooked with beef stock, I'm not going to touch it. Even if it means skipping a meal. But if I find out it was cooked with fish stock, chances are I will eat it. Maybe one day I'll evolve to a space where I won't even do that, but for now that's how I'm living. And I'm cool with it. Find a similar space and then make yourself comfortable there.

Ultimately, what's most important is that you're grateful for your meal. If you end up eating a side of rice with some spinach while all your friends dig into steaks, don't feel like your night was ruined—even if they ask you to chip in on the bill at the end of the night! Be happy in the knowledge that you made a compassionate choice.

EATING AT FRIENDS' WITHOUT BEING A PAIN

Telling a waiter politely—but firmly—that you'd like a dish prepared without meat or dairy is one thing. But telling a relative or a friend that you'd like a vegan or vegetarian option when you come over for dinner can be a much more stressful conversation. So I want to share some final tips on how to make sure that your diet doesn't become an issue between you and your friends and family.

Chances are you will experience a range of responses to your food choices. Some will be very accepting, whereas others will be downright adversarial. You're going to have some who will enjoy helping you come up with some vegan options. You'll have others who will go to great lengths to express concern that you're not getting enough protein or nutrients (even though they themselves may not have had a green vegetable in weeks).

Whatever the case may be, here are a couple of strategies that will help ensure you'll have lots of good food to eat and little or no drama:

• Always call ahead and offer to bring your own dish. Some people tend to get nervous and uptight when they entertain. The idea of having to cook a vegan dish they're unfamiliar with on top of what they were already planning might put them over the edge. Instead of stressing them out, just tell them you'll bring your own plate. Sometimes even just offering will put them at ease, and they'll happily make you a salad or pasta instead.

• Offer to chip in for ingredients if they do end up cooking a vegan or vegetarian dish especially for you. Chances are they'll tell you not to worry about it, but the gesture will be appreciated.

• Don't assume whomever you're visiting knows what being a vegan entails. A friend or relative might serve you eggs or dairy and truly believe that they made you a vegan meal. When you call ahead, just casually mention, "I'm vegan—that means no meat, fish, eggs, or dairy products."

- If you're hosting the party or holiday dinner, let everyone in advance know that you're going to be serving a vegan meal. And just as you might have brought a vegan meal to a dinner at their home, extend the same courtesy to them. Let them know if they're not interested in trying your food, they'll be missing out on a good meal, but they're welcome to bring their own dish.

You might not like the idea of animal products being eaten in your house. I certainly don't. I have people stay with me all the time, but if they want to eat any animal products, I ask them to keep it in a little fridge I have set up in my guesthouse. Part of me would rather ban animal products completely, but I believe it's better to keep a friendship alive than to make someone uncomfortable in my home. The longer you and that person are friends, the greater the chance they'll be inspired by your example and eventually stop eating animal products themselves.

- Don't get into a fight over food. If people ask questions about your diet, answer them as honestly as you can. If they tease you, throw a joke right back at them. If they try to provoke you into an argument, don't take the bait. Remember, people who feel threatened by your compassionate choice most likely are dealing with some sort of hurt themselves. Again, try to treat their pain with the same compassion you feel for animals' pain. Even if you feel like you're under attack.

Ultimately your best argument for going vegan can't be expressed in words anyway. It's going to be your happy aura. Your glowing skin. Your slim figure. Your wellness. Your peacefulness.

The type of beautiful energy that makes someone think, "I want some of that peace and wellness for myself."

TALKING TO YOUR DOCTOR

As discussed, when you begin to transition out of eating animal products, it's probably a good idea to go see a doctor and discuss any underlying health issues you might have, including checking for a vitamin B_{12} deficiency.

But be warned—there are doctors out there who will try to talk you out of going vegan. Not because that's what the latest research suggests or even because they have any firsthand experience with patients who don't eat animal products. But rather because they simply aren't as informed as they should be.

For every Dr. Ornish who saved Bill Clinton's life by suggesting he become a vegan, there are many more who unwittingly dissuade their patients from making the same change. According to surveys, on average most medical students receive less than twenty-four hours of nutrition training during their four years at medical school. Sorry, but a lot of those doctors don't know shit when it comes to what you should be putting in your body.

It's a real problem, because it can be confusing and anxiety producing to have a doctor question why you're not eating animal products. We're raised to trust our doctors and take their word as law when it comes to our health. But no matter how well intentioned they may be, doctors are not nutritionists, and when it comes to food they can be just as subjective as we are.

Sometimes it's not ignorance. There are doctors whose judgment is compromised by being on the payroll of pharmaceutical companies. Even if they know that going to a plant-based diet is the best treatment for your high blood pressure, they'll prescribe pills anyway. If you're curious just how much your doctors receive—in the form of payments, free meals, or trips—from pharmaceutical companies, enter their info at projects.propublica.org/docdollars. What you find might explain why your doctor seems a lot more interested in getting you on a certain medication than on having you change your diet.

Instead of relying solely on a doctor, consult with a licensed nutritionist as well. Nutritionists and dietitians are generally well versed in the benefits of vegetarian diets. The American Dietetic Association recently released a statement recommending vegetarian diets: "It is the position of the American Dietetic Association that appropriately planned vegetarian diets, including total vegetarian or vegan diets, are healthful, nutritionally adequate, and may provide health benefits in the prevention and treatment of certain diseases." They went on to say, "Well-planned vegetarian diets are appropriate for individuals during all stages of the lifecycle, including pregnancy, lactation, infancy, childhood, and adolescence, and for athletes."

You can find a list of nutritionists who specialize in vegan and vegetarian diets at Vegetarian Nutrition (vegetariannutrition.net/rd).

A doctor can write you a prescription for a lot of conditions, but happiness is one thing she doesn't have a script for. Happiness can't be swallowed in a pill, sprayed through an inhaler, or rubbed on in a cream. Happiness can only come through service and sacrifice. That's it.

This is not the message we usually hear. We're usually told that happiness comes from love. But as painful as it might be to admit, we all know that love is not something we can hold on to long-term. Love, we learn again and again, is often fleeting.

Even more often, we're told that happiness comes from worldly success. We're taught that making a lot of money, buying a new car, being given an award, or going on a vacation will bring joy to our lives. While those are all fun things to experience, they only represent what I call "short-term happiness." You are not going to experience lasting happiness from riding around in a new car or sitting on a beach for a few days. And when you make the mistake of confusing short-term happiness for lasting happiness, it can become very depressing.

Lasting happiness requires work. It requires courage. It requires commitment. You must accept the simple fact that you can't be happy and hurtful at the same time. It's impossible. When you're hurting yourself, hurting animals, and hurting Mother Earth through your diet, your soul is never going to feel right. But if you put in even just a little bit of work and begin to cut animal products out of your diet, you'll start to feel better about things. If you make a commitment to that process and eventually cut all that suffering out of your diet, you'll feel great. And if you have the courage to stand by that decision, even when other people don't understand or support it, in short time you will feel content, energized, and, yes, happy—in a way you probably haven't experienced before.

That's why I called this book *The Happy Vegan*.

Because when you're committed to not only saving animals and the earth but also saving *yourself*, happiness is inevitable.

The work and commitment required won't go away. I've been practicing this lifestyle for almost twenty years and there are still moments when I wake up and don't feel like meditating, but I stay committed to the practice and afterward I feel great. Just as there are still plenty of afternoons when I'm tired and dragging and don't really want to go to yoga, but I remind myself that it's important to me. And when I walk out of the class, I feel as light as a feather. Just as there are still plenty of times I'll see someone eating a chicken wing and think, "Just one bite wouldn't be so bad." But I resist that temptation because I know when I contribute to the suffering of another being—even just one bite—it's going to be at the expense of my happiness.

So as you leave these pages and move back out into the world, please try to carry this simple message with you: Happiness is addictive.

Right now, you might be addicted to any number of things, from the high of drugs to the taste of fat and salt. But I promise that if you can make the "sacrifice" to remove those harmful, negative influences from your life, the world is going to open up in front of you. A path that might seem to be filled with obstacles is suddenly going to look like an open highway.

You are going to see that the long-term happiness that might have seemed so elusive has been within your grasp all along. All you need is the courage to reach and grab it.

ADDITIONAL RESOURCES

WEBSITES

happycow.com: HappyCow was created as a public service to assist travelers and people everywhere in finding vegan, vegetarian, and healthy food. It's no surprise that this is my go-to site when I'm on the road. Simply type the city or region you're headed to and HappyCow's search engine will give you a list of vegan, vegetarian, and vegan-friendly restaurants in that area. They've also got a detailed database for when you are traveling internationally.

peta.com: Lots of helpful tips, information, and inspiration. One especially cool thing they'll do is hook you up with a "vegan mentor" if you feel you need somebody to support you through the process of giving up animal products.

vegnews.com: When I want to explore with a new food or just need to remotivate myself about all the wonderful food choices out there, I head to VegNews. Tons of delicious recipes as well as travel tips. They also have job listings for positions within the vegan community.

latestvegannews.com: As its name suggests, Latest Vegan News is a great site to keep you updated on everything affecting vegans. From the latest medical benefits to giving up animal products to what celebrity just landed a vegan cooking show, this site has it all.

thisrawsomeveganlife.com: This Rawsome Vegan Life offers tons of delicious recipes and lifestyle tips, with an emphasis on raw foods.

sistahvegan.com: The Sistah Vegan Project is a great resource for those trying to build a sense of community, especially for African American women. The site's founder and editor, A. Breeze Harper, has created a space that speaks directly to some of the issues people of color in particular will experience when they give up animal products. She also has some really great advice on cooking with kids.

garden-of-vegan.tumblr.com: Check out Garden of Vegan, a Tumblr blog with beautiful photos of delicious vegan meals. The site includes hundreds of yummy recipes, with a really helpful section with ideas for on-the-go snacks.

ohsheglows.com: The Oh She Glows website has over five hundred vegan recipes, many of which are gluten-free. Going gluten-free and vegan can seem intimidating, so definitely check out this site if that's something you're facing. The site also has some very useful tips on what to buy for your kitchen when you first begin your vegan journey.

RECOMMENDED COOKBOOKS

When I first began working on this book my plan was to include some recipes from some of the vegan chefs who have worked with me over the years.

But as I began to compile a list, the process felt kind of disingenuous to me. It wasn't that they hadn't cooked some delicious meals for me—they certainly had!

I think I felt a little uneasy because at the end of the day, I'm not a chef myself. Not only that, I barely cook a thing. Sometimes I'll sauté a little spinach with crushed red peppers, but truthfully that's about it. I'm not proud of the fact I don't cook much, and it's something I need to work on. But as it stands right now, I'm not a cook and it doesn't feel right trying to share "my" recipes.

Having said that, I don't want to sell you on the concept of a plant-based diet but then leave you without any resources on how to prepare it. So I called around to some of my vegan friends who spend a little bit more time in the kitchen than I do and found out what books they recommend.

What follows is a list of cookbooks that my friends and colleagues say are the among the easiest and most accessible introductions to a plant-based diet. I hope the recipes in these books will become staples of your new diet and that you'll enjoy these meals in health and happiness.

Gannon, Sharon. *Simple Recipes for Joy: More Than 200 Delicious Vegan Recipes.* New York: Avery, 2014.

Holloway, Matt, and Michelle Davis. *Thug Kitchen: Eat Like You Give a F*ck.* New York: Rodale Books, 2014.

Liddon, Angela. *The Oh She Glows Cookbook: Over 100 Vegan Recipes to Glow from the Inside Out.* New York: Avery, 2014.

Quivers, Robin. *The Vegucation of Robin: How Real Food Saved My Life.* New York: Avery, 2013.

Roll, Rich, and Julie Piatt. *The Plantpower Way: Whole Food Plant-Based Recipes and Guidance for the Whole Family.* New York: Avery, 2015.

Sroufe, Del. *Forks Over Knives: The Cookbook: Over 300 Recipes for Plant-Based Eating All through the Year.* New York: The Experiment, 2012.

APPENDIX: A GUIDE TO MEDITATION

'm so thankful that after reading an entire book about the benefits of giving up animal products, you're still taking the time to learn something about the practice of meditation. As I said, I know from firsthand experience that meditation will completely transform your lifestyle and make your transition to a plant-based diet so much easier.

Now you might be thinking that something that changes your life in such a profound way must be pretty difficult to learn, right? Or you might be asking, Won't I need a lot of fancy equipment or a special place to practice it?

Not at all.

All you need to meditate is twenty minutes and a comfortable place to sit. No high-tech machines, no special workout gear, no membership to a club. Just you, your mind, and a seat. It couldn't be any less complicated.

Despite its simplicity, meditation doesn't always seem like the most accessible practice to novices. The idea of sitting in silence for twenty minutes can actually seem quite intimidating to some people. In order to help you get past any misconceptions or fears you might have about the process, I'd like to walk you through the practice of meditation, in terms of what you will experience both physically and mentally as you move out of the distractions of the world and into a restful state of deep consciousness.

I both practice and promote a *mantra-based form of meditation*, which involves repeating a sound in your head for twenty minutes. It's a style of meditation that I've learned from several sources, including Sharon Gannon and my great friend Bob Roth, who teaches Transcendental Meditation through the David Lynch Foundation. The organization does incredible work helping spread the word about how meditation can change not only lives but also the world. What I'm about to teach you incorporates elements of what I learned from both Sharon and Bob, as well as other masters that I've studied with during my travels around the world. It's the style I've promoted in *Super Rich* and *Success Through Stillness*, and almost every day I'm stopped by someone on the street who tells me learning how to meditate through those books transformed their lives.

YOUR SEAT

To begin, the first thing you should do is find a quiet place where you can sit comfortably for those twenty minutes. Unless you live out in the country somewhere, chances are you won't be able to find a completely quiet place, but that's fine. You might hear a bit of traffic, a dog barking, maybe kids playing in the next apartment, but don't let that discourage you. A couple of minutes into your practice, you won't notice any of those sounds. And if you feel like they're truly going to keep distracting you, try this trick: Bring a couple of the pillows into the bathroom with you. That's the one place in your house that you can usually count on to be pretty quiet. Put the toilet seat down and sit on it, with one pillow underneath you and another behind you. You'll be comfortable that way and won't hear too many noises.

Once you've found a good spot, sit in whatever manner seems the most comfortable to you. If you want to sit in the traditional Lotus Pose, with legs crossed in front of you and hands resting upturned on your thighs, that's fine. If you want to sit in a comfortable chair, that's fine too. If you want to sit on something more rigid, like a kitchen or folding chair, that will work too. Whatever kind of seat you choose, just try to keep your back as straight and your posture as upright as possible. Try to think of there being a string that someone's pulling on that runs from the top of your head all the way up to heaven. Even if you can't maintain that sort of erect posture throughout your practice, you want to get in the habit of not slouching too much.

Once you've settled into your seat, go through this quick checklist to make sure the rest of your body is in proper alignment:

- **Hands.** Make sure they're relaxed. If you're in a chair, you can just lay them flat on your thighs. If you're in the Lotus Pose, you can do the same thing, just with your palms up on your thighs.
- **Shoulders.** Roll them a few times to make sure you're not holding any tension in them and then let them relax.
- **Your head.** Pull back your chin so that your head is perfectly aligned with your spine. It will feel like you're giving yourself a

double chin, but that's fine. Then imagine a piece of string running from the base of your spine up through the top of your head and then all the way into the heavens. If that string feels slack or loose, then you're not doing it right. But if that imaginary string seems taut, like you're hanging from a hook in the sky, then you've got it.

- **Tongue.** Let it rest gently against the back of your top teeth. This will keep your mouth from becoming too dry while you meditate.

Now you're ready for your mantra.

YOUR MANTRA

If you're not familiar with the term, a *mantra* refers to a sound or vibration that you'll repeat through your practice. Even though many mantras are based on ancient Hindu words, don't think of yours as having any meaning while you meditate.

While some people have their mantra assigned to them by a master based on their age and personality, the mantra I'm going to share with you here is a mass mantra, one that is appropriate for people of any age. It was taught to me by a master who said it has been used by a wide range of people for over a thousand years.

And the mantra is *rum*.

Now when you read the word *rum* on the page, you might be tempted to assign a meaning to it. Most likely the alcohol. But please let go of whatever sort of association the word might conjure in your mind. In fact, don't think if it as a word at all. Think of it as nothing more than a sound or vibration.

Now that you've detached any meaning from the word, try saying it:

Rum.

Next, say it silently in your mind, even stretching it out a little bit.

Ruuuuuuum.

Then say it fast:

RumRumRumRum.

Say it over and over again in your mind, in as many different ways as possible, until you feel completely at ease. So that instead of being a word, it feels like just another part of your body.

After about thirty seconds of playing around with the sound, gently close your eyes. Your meditation has begun.

When you begin repeating *rum*, you might be aware of the thoughts coming in and out of your mind. Don't let that discourage you. The point of meditation, despite what some people think, is not to turn off your mind. Rather, you're simply looking to detach yourself from those thoughts.

Think of the thoughts coming in and out of your mind as the waves on a stormy ocean. The more you keep repeating *rum* to yourself, the stronger its vibration will become. As the vibration grows stronger, the waves will become smaller and smaller, until in time you will barely notice them at all. When that happens, you will be in a space of pure stillness.

Despite your best efforts to find a quiet, secluded spot, distractions might occur. A car alarm might go off on your street. Your neighbor might start playing his music loud. Your nose might start to itch.

Whatever the case may be, don't try to fight that distraction. If you hear a loud noise, acknowledge it and gently return to your mantra. If your nose is itching like crazy, scratch it and then gently return to your mantra.

What you'll find is that the deeper you get into your meditation, the less and less you'll be distracted by outside elements. To the point where someone could be banging on the door of the room you're in and you wouldn't even notice it. That's because the deeper you go into stillness, the better it feels. You'll feel so at peace that you won't want to move an inch if it means disturbing that tranquility.

Even if it doesn't always feel like it, our mind's natural inclination is to go to the most peaceful, restful place possible. Just as water always runs downstream, our minds always seek out a tranquil place. If you learn anything from meditation, let it be that peacefulness and restfulness is actually your natural state. By letting your mind get caught up in the distractions of life, you've essentially been asking water to run upstream. Which is why life can often feel like an uphill battle. Meditation will teach you how to detach yourself from those distractions and let the water of your spirit follow its natural course again, away from the noise and into your heart.

YOUR THOUGHTS

Don't be alarmed if after repeating *rum* for several minutes a thought reenters your head. It could be about something you forgot to do at work or a conversation you were having with your boyfriend the night before. Whatever the case might be, don't get frustrated. Or even worse, open your eyes and quit your practice. Simply consider it for a moment and then gently return to your mantra. Don't try to fight it or push it out of your mind. Just stay committed to your mantra and eventually that thought will drift out of your mind, like a leaf being carried along the surface of a rolling stream.

To better understand this process, think of your mind as a cage and your thoughts as a monkey. When you first sit down in your seat and begin to repeat *rum* that monkey might start acting a fool. Banging on its chest, swinging around the cage, making loud monkey sounds. Doing anything it can to throw you off your game.

But if you just sit back and chill while repeating your mantra, eventually the monkey is going to lose interest. Instead of banging on its cage, it's going wander off and stop making noise. It might take a couple of minutes for that monkey to lose interest, but it will. Remember, your mantra is always going to beat that monkey.

To really hammer this concept home, let me offer a final analogy. Have you ever slept next to an old-fashioned alarm clock? The kind that literally goes *tick-tock-tick*? If you have, then you know that when you first lay down to sleep that ticking can sound awfully loud. To the point where you might think to yourself, "Man, it's going to be impossible for me to fall asleep with this shit ticking in my ear."

Yet despite how loud it might sound at first, as you lay in bed and your mind begins to settle, the ticking won't bother you anymore. Before long you can't even hear it at all and you drift off to sleep.

That ticking noise never actually went away. Its volume was just as loud when you first lay down as when you eventually fell asleep. It's just that as you became more restful, your mind flowed away from the distraction of the ticking and toward the peace of stillness.

When you meditate, your thoughts will be like the ticking of the alarm clock. They're never going to disappear, but the more peaceful and restful you become, the less and less you'll be aware of them.

TAKING INVENTORY

Once that monkey goes away, you'll be in the first stage of meditation, which is known as "quieter thought." Or as I like to call it, "taking inventory." During this stage, any thought that enters your mind will appear slowly and peacefully. Instead of a monkey swinging on the bars of a cage, imagine a swan gliding serenely across a pond.

Many of my best ideas have come to me during this stage. This is because as you sink deeper into stillness, all the junk that's accumulated in your mind begins to fade away, leaving only your good thoughts. Your pure thoughts. Your highest thoughts.

The thoughts that reflect how you *truly* feel, instead of what the world has told you to feel. These are the thoughts that are going to show you the right decision to make in your career. In your personal life. And with the world.

If you have a moment, as I'm sure you will, when you suddenly think, "I don't want to eat animal products anymore," it's going to come during this stage. Because instead of hearing all the noise about why meat is OK or natural, all you're going to hear is your body telling you that it doesn't feel good when you eat meat. Just as you're going to hear your soul telling you to detach yourself from the suffering of the animals.

It's very important to take your time and not rush through this stage. You want to consider these pure thoughts very slowly. Not every one of them is going to make you a million dollars or even make you give up animal products that very day. However, when you get in the practice of spending time in this inventory stage every single day, you will become much more familiar with your true self. So that over time, instead of getting entangled in the distraction of the world, you will start to develop a much greater sense of clarity. Clarity about your relationships, your lifestyle, and your connection to the world.

PURE CONSCIOUSNESS

After a few minutes of taking inventory, you will begin to enter what I call the stage of "pure consciousness." This is where your thoughts finally give way to your mantra, and you can access the limitless pool of stillness inside of you.

Bob Roth describes pure consciousness this way: Think of your mind as being like the ocean. On the surface of the ocean it's choppy and there are a lot of waves. That's your distracted mind.

But at the bottom of the ocean, it's still. That's your mind in a state of pure consciousness.

Despite the absence of thought, pure consciousness is where some of your greatest ideas will come to you. The director David Lynch, who works with Bob at promoting meditation, has a great way to describe this concept. "Ideas are like fish," he says. "If you want to catch little fish, you can stay in the shallow water. But if you want to catch the big fish, you've got to go deeper. Down deep, the fish are more powerful and more pure. They're huge and abstract. And they're beautiful."

Not only is pure consciousness the stage where you'll be able to land the big fish that have been swimming around in your mind but it's also the stage that promotes the physical healing that comes through meditation.

While you don't necessarily want to fall asleep while you meditate (if you do happen to, just return to your mantra when you wake up) the rest you receive during this stage will be very beneficial. Studies have shown that the rest you'll experience is as deep or even deeper than what you might experience during nightly sleep.

Studies have also shown that detaching yourself from your thoughts is extremely beneficial for your nervous system. Thoughts (at least distracted ones) often lead to stress, which in turn leads to a host of conditions like high blood pressure and stroke. This is why people who practice meditation are 30 percent less likely to die from heart disease than the general population. No wonder insurance companies have started offering reimbursements to people who meditate.

ENDING YOUR SESSION

OK, you've been sitting comfortably in your seat, back and head as straight as possible, repeating *rum*. You let the monkey quiet down, took inventory, and then slowly drifted into a state of pure consciousness. Maybe you even caught a big fish!

So how do you know that your twenty minutes are up if you're in a state of pure consciousness?

I've found the easiest way is to set the timer on my smartphone for twenty minutes right before I begin repeating my mantra. I strongly suggest you put your phone on low volume and gentle alarm because even then it's going to sound extremely loud when it goes off. I know that if I'm meditating with a friend and he coughs or just clears his throat, it feels like a bomb went off. This is because your sense of sound is extremely heightened during pure consciousness.

Whatever you do, you don't want to have a jarring sound signal the end of your twenty minutes. It's critical that when your time is over, you slowly ease yourself out of pure consciousness and back into the world. Otherwise there's a strong chance you won't be able to hold on to some of those pure thoughts you encountered during your session.

Despite the possibility of a jarring reentry into the world, I recommend a timer for beginners because otherwise they're likely to be distracted by worrying about whether they've been meditating long enough.

It's not uncommon for beginners to get stuck on thoughts about how long they've been meditating, where they ask themselves over and over again, "Hasn't it been twenty minutes yet? I feel like I've been doing this for a long time." When that happens, it can become tempting to open your eyes and check the clock. Which of course makes it much harder for you to slip into that state of pure consciousness.

But if you set your timer and press start, you won't have to worry about constantly checking the time. Even though there may be moments when it feels like you've been going for way more than twenty minutes, until you hear that buzzer, you won't get entangled in those thoughts.

Even after the buzzer sounds, I still recommend that you spend a minimum of one minute sitting with your eyes closed, slowly letting your mantra fade out of your mind. Don't worry if you're not sure exactly when a minute or two has passed: Your body will let you know when it's ready for you to open your eyes again.

WALKING MEDITATION

When you finally do open your eyes and reenter the world, you'll feel a difference immediately. The feeling isn't the same every time, but you'll always feel better than you did before you started meditating.

It's certainly true on a physical level. If you woke up in the morning with a stuffy nose, you're going to be breathing better. If you woke up with a headache, you're going to feel clearheaded. If you woke up feeling stressed about the day ahead of you, after twenty minutes you'll have a hard time remembering why you were wound so tightly.

Though it might not happen every day, there are going to be times when you come out of your practice, and it will feel like you're reentering a different world. And for the better. When you open your eyes, the room might appear brighter and prettier than it did before. Colors will seem more vivid and alive. You'll notice the birds chirping outside and appreciate their beautiful melodies. You might even start giggling. I certainly have.

This is why it's critical you don't rush back into your normal routine. Don't grab your phone and check to see who e-mailed you during your meditation. Or immediately turn on the TV. Try to take that feeling of peace and happiness and extend it as long as possible.

When you carry that energy with you out of your meditation and into your day, you'll be entering a state of what I call "walking meditation." It might last only an hour or two before the feeling starts to fade, but it's still an amazing experience for even that short amount of time. When you get a glimpse of how you could be living your entire life, it's going to inspire you to become even more dedicated to your practice.

Walking meditation is going to be what gives you the clarity to make better choices when it comes your lifestyle. You might have the big moment of "I don't want to eat animal products anymore" during pure consciousness, but it's walking meditation that will allow you to apply that decision to your day-to-day life.

When you're in a state of walking meditation, if you pick up some chicken wings at the store, you'll be able to look past the idyllic farm on the package and see through to the suffering those birds were put through. When you're in walking meditation, you're going to be able to feel the stress animal products put on your body. When you're in walking meditation, you're going to be able to draw a very clear line between the meat and dairy industries and the damage being done to our environment. And because your mind will be so clear and free of distractions, you'll be able to make the right choices with that information.

Please just remember that walking meditation doesn't happen after just one or two practices. To live in this state, you must make the meditation a permanent part of your lifestyle.

It might feel like a grind at first, but if you are patient with the process, eventually the change in you will become permanent. You'll hear less and less noise from the world and more of your best ideas. This is why it's so important to practice meditation *religiously*. As I always say, you're not going to get muscles from one push-up. Just as you're not going to lose twenty pounds just by skipping one meal.

In order to achieve lasting happiness, you must make a real commitment to this process.

I am not saying that it's impossible to become a vegan without also being a meditator. There might be some readers who made the decision to give up animal products before they even got to this section.

But if you're still on the fence or are harboring any nagging doubts about whether you can do it, then please make a commitment to meditation.

The worst-case scenario is that after sitting in silence once a day for several weeks you'll reduce your stress and lower your blood pressure. In the unlikely event you take nothing else from the practice, lowering your stress is guaranteed.

It's much more likely, however, that through meditation you will find yourself tapping a source of both strength and serenity you might not have known you possessed. A source of peacefulness will empower you to make the best choices for both your mind and your spirit. That will empower you to reject poison and choose healing. That will empower you to stop contributing to one of the greatest problems in the world and become part of the solution instead.

Your whole life is nothing but a journey toward discovering these truths within yourself. Don't wait any longer. Embrace the stillness in your heart and start that journey today.

ACKNOWLEDGMENTS

I want to thank some of the heroes of the animal rights movement: Ingrid Newkirk of PETA, Nathan Runkle of Mercy For Animals, Gene Baur of Farm Sanctuary, my great friend Simone Reyes, plus so many other brave individuals and groups who are fighting the good fight against animal cruelty. I also want to acknowledge physicians like Dr. Colin Campbell, Dr. Caldwell B. Esselstyn, and Dr. Dean Ornish, whose writings and research have done so much to awaken the public to the grave dangers associated with eating animal products.